ALOE

VERA

ALOE VERA

Nature's Soothing Healer

DIANE GAGE

Healing Arts Press
Rochester, Vermont

Healing Arts Press
One Park Street
Rochester, Vermont 05767
www.InnerTraditions.com

Note to the reader: *This book is intended as an informational guide. The
remedies, approaches, and techniques described herein are meant to supplement, and not to be a substitute for, professional medical care or treatment.
They should not be used to treat a serious ailment without prior consultation
with a qualified healthcare professional.*

LIBRARY OF CONGRESS CATALOGING-IN-PUBLICATION DATA

Gage, Diane.
    Aloe vera : nature's soothing healer / Diane Gage.
      p. cm.
    Includes bibliographical references (p.).
    ISBN 0-89281-627-9
    1. Aloe barbadensis—Therapeutic use. 2. Aloe barbadensis. 3. Subject C.
I. Title.
RM666.A414G33 1996
615'.324324–dc20   95-43957
                                         CIP

Printed and bound in Canada

10 9 8 7 6 5 4 3

Text design and layout by Charlotte Tyler
This book was typeset in Italian Electric

Healing Arts Press is a division of Inner Traditions International

Contents

Acknowledgments

My sincere thanks to the following individuals who gave of their time, talent, friendship, and love to help me research and write this book: Sue Leibovitz Schudson, Vicki Townsend Gibbs, Pat Rarus, Charlotte Coleman, Laurie Taylor-Donald, Suzanne Jackson, Noonie Benford, and Gene Gage, Jr.

I would also like to thank my agent Bill Gladstone, president of Waterside Productions, for suggesting this project to me, and Ehud Sperling and Leslie Colket of Healing Arts Press for seeing the need for this book.

A special note of appreciation goes to the aloe vera growers, manufacturers, distributors, and consumers. The information and experiences they shared with me greatly facilitated the writing of this book and have made it a better resource for those who want to learn about aloe vera.

PREFACE

This book is intended to introduce you to aloe vera so that you may make your own decision about how and whether the plant might be beneficial to you. Each chapter contains opinions about and testimonials to aloe vera's efficacy and reports on aloe vera research. As you read, you'll see some contradictory comments. That is a reflection of the diversity of public opinion: some people have seen remarkable results from using the aloe vera plant and aloe vera-based products, while others are more skeptical about its usefulness.

Each year more research is being done on the effectiveness of aloe vera, but much more needs to be done before aloe vera is fully accepted by the medical and scientific communities and, in turn, the consumer. While scientific research and clinical substantiation may be slow in coming, the personal testimonials from people who have benefited in some way from using this plant are plentiful. Distributors of aloe vera—although they emphasize that they make no medical claims for their products—are eager to share reports of the many ways aloe vera has been used to cure every kind of problem from psoriasis to stomach ulcers and skin cancer.

Although usually slow to endorse new treatments, the

medical community does not completely turn a deaf ear to such testimonials. One reason is that many physicians have themselves seen their patients benefit from using aloe vera. And some physicians have incorporated the use of aloe vera into their practices and their personal lives.

Before you read further, a word of caution is necessary. Those who use aloe vera regularly and those who grow, manufacture, and sell it know that aloe vera has limitations. It is not a cure-all, as some people have professed in the past.

If you decide to use aloe vera or aloe vera products to treat an illness or injury, don't ignore the opinions of medical specialists. As with any product, read the instructions carefully and use aloe vera in moderation.

On occasion, specific names of products have been included in this book at the request of those who shared their testimonials and are not meant as an endorsement. The companies and brands mentioned here are only a sampling of the aloe vera industry and its many products.

ALOE VERA COMES OF AGE 1

To many people aloe vera is simply a folk remedy, used for the quick relief of minor cuts and burns, while to others it's a decorative houseplant. To some, it's the latest wonder in "natural" ingredients.

Aloe vera is this and more: it is the basis of a multi-million dollar industry of dietary and health supplements, beauty aids, and pharmaceutical creams. Not only that, it has captured the interest of scientists and medical researchers throughout the world who are working to discover and identify the source of the healing properties of the soothing gel and translucent juice stored inside its leaves.

Crucial discoveries in recent years have brought scientists even closer to identifying the source of the healing properties within the soothing gel and translucent juice stored inside the aloe vera plant's leaves. Studies have revealed that one of several active ingredients is a complex carbohydrate called acemannan. Such new information has opened the doors for potential new applications and uses of aloe's healing abilities in the treatment of cancers, tumors, ulcers, wounds, inflammatory diseases, and, most significantly, infectious diseases such as HIV and AIDS.

In more traditional uses, physicians use aloe vera–based creams to heal serious thermal injuries, such as burns and frostbite. Dentists employ aloe vera gels to reduce swelling and inflammation of the gums. Dermatologists rely on aloe vera products to help clear acne, and optometrists find the products helpful in soothing eye inflammations. Professional sports trainers treat their athletes' muscle aches and sprains, skin abrasions, and blisters with aloe vera products. Cosmetics companies incorporate aloe vera into skin creams, soaps, and shampoos, not only for the beneficial effects aloe vera is said to have on the skin and hair but also for the marketing appeal the words "made with aloe" now have for the consumer. Drinking aloe vera juice is said to have therapeutic effects on arthritis, ulcers, diabetes, and other health conditions. The wide range of applications, and the beneficial effects of its use, continue to increase the popularity of this ancient plant.

THE ALOE PLANT

There are over 275 species in the genus *Aloe* worldwide. Of the three to four species used commercially, the most popular is *Aloe barbadensis* Miller (also known as *Aloe vera* Linne, *Aloe vulgaris* Lamarck, and other names), most commonly called aloe vera.

The name *aloe vera*, Latin for "true aloe," was probably given to this particular plant because it is the aloe species reputed to be the most medicinally beneficial and therapeutic. It is also the most widely available species of the medicinal aloes and the only one cultivated in the western hemisphere.

Today, the plant is grown in India, China, South and Central America, the Caribbean, Spain, Mexico, North America—primarily Texas and Florida—and other tropical and semitropical regions.

Its thick, thorn-edged leaves, ranging in color from grey to bright green, give aloe vera the appearance of a cactus, but it is, in fact, a member of the lily family *(Liliaceae)*. Cousin to the onion, garlic, asparagus, and turnip, aloe's relationship to the lily becomes apparent when the plant blooms. A typical aloe vera plant produces two or three yellow tubular flowers, shaped much like those of the Easter Lily, and it flowers intermittently throughout the year.

The dagger-shaped aloe vera leaves grow from the base of the plant in a rosette pattern. Full-grown plants range in size from one and a half to four feet tall and have an average of fifteen leaves. The leaves of a mature aloe vera plant measure about three or more inches across at the base and weigh from one to three pounds each. Depending on weather and soil conditions, the plant reaches maturity in one and a half to five years. Many aloe growers and product manufacturers warn that immature aloe vera plants, often including many household potted plants, do not have the same chemical potency as a mature plant.

The word *aloe* is derived from the Arabic *alloeh* or the Hebrew *halal,* meaning "bitter, shiny substance"—a description that fits only one of two distinct materials found in the aloe vera leaf. Located in a corrugated lining immediately beneath the inner surface of the plant's skin is the latex, commonly called the yellow sap. The sap, which is bitter to the taste and irritates the lips, and the thorny edges of the leaves are thought to deter animals and insects from eating the plant.

The latex, when dried and powdered, has been used as a laxative by many cultures. The Arabs first recorded using aloe vera as a laxative during the sixth century B.C. Later, the plant was grown and harvested for its yellow sap in the Caribbean Islands, primarily in Barbados. Because biologists of the seventeenth century thought, erroneously, that the plant was native to the island, they coined aloe vera's botanical name *barbadensis*.

As more reliable laxatives were made, the use of aloe vera sap diminished because its cathartic effects were often unreliable and sometimes violent. Today, the latex of the aloe vera plant is still recognized as a drug by the United States' official drug compendium, the *U. S. Pharmacopoeia*. According to Emil Corwin, Information Officer for the United States Food and Drug Administration (FDA), over-the-counter drugs containing aloe vera continue to be sold. The FDA says, however, that medical sources, including the American Medical Association and the American Pharmaceutical Association, recommend that aloe vera not be used as a laxative because it can cause intestinal griping and cramping.

The other major part of the aloe vera leaf, the clear, semi-solid substance that makes up the parenchyma, is known as the gel. The gel has a distinct vegetable odor, considered unpleasant by some people. It is the aloe vera gel that enables the plant to hold moisture for extremely long periods of time. As a member of the botanical class Xerophytes (to which such plants as the cactus, agave and yucca belong), aloe vera has the ability to completely close its stomata to avoid water loss and survive long periods of time without water. For the same reason, if a leaf is cut, the wound heals quickly and the plant grows in another direction.

Although generally not recognized as a drug by the FDA,

the gel of the aloe vera plant has been used for centuries to heal burns, cuts, and skin irritations and to soften and moisten skin. According to the FDA, there has not been enough scientific evidence to prove the plant's effectiveness in treating minor skin conditions, yet people continue to report remarkable results from the topical application of aloe vera.

Although the FDA cannot require cosmetics manufacturers to test the safety of their products before they are marketed, it reports no problems with cosmetics containing aloe vera.

Many people use aloe vera gel or juice as a dietary supplement (aloe vera juice is an extract of aloe vera gel, but the terms gel and juice are used synonymously throughout the aloe vera industry; see Appendix A for a definition). Some drink it primarily to regulate elimination, while others claim it gives them more energy. Still other people drink aloe vera to treat a variety of health conditions, such as arthritis, diabetes, ulcers, or indigestion. According to the FDA, no conclusive scientific studies have been done to determine the benefits or drawbacks of drinking a daily dose of aloe vera.

Nevertheless, the widely held belief in the curative properties of the plant's gel has earned aloe vera such nicknames as "the medical plant," "the wand of heaven," and "the potted physician." Indeed, the folklore behind the plant's healing and moisturizing properties has contributed to its popularity.

FOLKLORE HAS ITS PLACE

While some people find little credibility in folklore, others contend that the legends that have followed aloe vera throughout the centuries add to the plant's credibility and should not be dismissed.

"Folk medicine is really a time test," says Robert Trotter II,

Ph.D., a medical anthropologist at Northern Arizona University in Flagstaff, Arizona. "In fact," he says, "studying folklore is one way scientists discover new medicines. If a plant has been used for the same thing for generations by different cultures which have had no contact, there's a good indication that the plant is an effective medicine. And that's what has happened with aloe vera."

Juan Antonio Chavira, Ph.D., J.D., of San Antonio, Texas, agrees: "Most folk medicine traditions that survive are ones that continue to benefit people. Aloe vera is still used today because people believe in its effectiveness and are satisfied with the results they've seen."

Aloe vera's ability to treat certain conditions is not just rooted in folklore however; the plant has a powerful biochemistry. "Historically, the aloe vera plant has been effective in treating minor burns—including sunburn—diabetes, ulcers, arthritis, and a wide variety of other conditions," says Dr. Trotter. "But because many aloe vera companies cannot afford to conduct the research necessary to prove the claims made about the plant, there is little evidence to support aloe vera's healing abilities.

"Aloe vera, like other plants, is not a controlled substance," Dr. Totter continues. "Consumers must gather enough information themselves about a product to make informed decisions on how to use it appropriately."

PUTTING ALOE TO USE

For centuries, the only way people could obtain aloe vera extracts was to cut open the leaf of the plant. It wasn't until the late 1960s with the development of methods for stabilizing aloe vera (preserving the plant in a way that retains the plant's biochemical activity), that gels and juices could be preserved, packaged and sold commercially.

Today, growing and selling aloe vera and its products is a multi-million dollar industry. Since the latest aloe boom began about two decades ago, as many claims have been made about its uses as there have been controversies about its effectiveness.

Although still used to heal burns, aloe vera is also frequently used as a topical application to treat skin abrasions, acne, athlete's foot, baldness, bruises, blisters, burns, dry skin, insect bites, muscle cramps, psoriasis, skin cancers and skin ulcers, and sunburn. Both the gel and the juice from the plant are taken internally to help cure such conditions as arthritis, bad breath, diabetes, headaches, high blood pressure, insomnia, and stomach ulcers.

Some use it as a deodorant or aftershave, and many find it as a prime ingredient in their soaps, shampoos, and facial and body creams. Some people say aloe vera rids pets of fleas.

It's because of this alphabet soup of claims and a lack of scientific evidence to support them that some consumers have become skeptical of the plant and its products. However, research and product testing is costly, and those who sell aloe vera products have been slow to develop scientific evidence to support the claims made for the plant.

Today, as aloe vera product sales increase, some companies in the United States, Japan, Germany, and Russia and other countries are conducting scientific research on the plant and its products and believe that their findings will help substantiate claims made about aloe vera.

Because most aloe vera manufacturers in the United States do not want to have their products regulated as drugs, few make therapeutic promises for their products. Instead, they depend on testimonials by the product distributors and consumers to prove the value of their aloe vera products.

Clinton Howard, founder of Carrington Laboratories, a Dallas-based manufacturer and distributor of aloe vera juice, skin care products, and pharmaceuticals, says that soon after his company began in 1974, reports on the medical benefits of his products began coming in. Most people who wrote were arthritis sufferers who claimed greater mobility and less pain and swelling once they started drinking aloe vera juice. Others wrote of good results from drinking the juice for a variety of gastrointestinal problems, while others found the gel effective in treating headaches, alleviating the itching from insect bites, and moisturizing dry skin and hair.

"At first, you don't pay much attention when you hear such claims, because there is a lot of subjective control over health," says Howard. "But when you hear the same claims hundreds of times, you begin to think that there might be something to them. We make aloe vera products because the public wants them, but we make no claims for their medical benefits."

Howard was intrigued enough by the claims made about his company's products, and pleased enough with the profit they generated, to hire pharmacologists and scientists to create a million-dollar laboratory where they could analyze the plant.

Carrington Laboratories is one of several companies studying aloe vera. Bill Coats, R.Ph., founder of Aloe Vera of America, the company that manufactures products distributed by Forever Living Products, is now the owner of Coats Aloe International, a company specializing in pharmaceutical and cosmetic uses of aloe vera. Coats says that his company employs BioSearch, a research laboratory in Dallas, to perform bacteriological studies on aloe vera products to determine how they react on human tissue. Coats, the author of *The Silent Healer: A Modern Study of Aloe Vera,* also works closely with dentists, dermatologists, athletic trainers, and veterinarians to study the effectiveness of his company's products.

"People don't believe in aloe vera products until they use them," says Coats. "The only skeptics I've met are people who have not used a properly stabilized aloe vera product. If a person with a painful ulcer feels relief within fifteen to twenty minutes of drinking two ounces of aloe vera juice, he's a believer in the product. And if a person with a bad sunburn is pain free minutes after she's been sprayed with aloe vera liquid, she becomes an advocate of aloe vera products, too."

Coats, a pharmacist by training, sold his five pharmacies to devote his time to the development of aloe vera products after he patented what he says was the first stabilization process for aloe vera in 1968. "Pharmacies can help people, but they are limited in scope," says Coats. "With aloe vera there is no limit to the amount of good that can be done.

"We live in a drug-oriented world, and while we need drugs, they can cause many side effects," Coats continues. "Our clinical studies have shown that people using aloe vera products can receive many of the same benefits as they get from drugs but without any of the reported contraindications."

Discerning the Truth

Despite the array of claims and the continual slow accretion of scientific evidence supporting aloe vera's effectiveness in treating burns, ulcers, and other health conditions, the FDA warns the public about exaggerated and unsubstantiated claims that aloe vera products can cure or alleviate a host of health problems.

Out of the controversy surrounding the plant and the competition among aloe vera growers, manufacturers, and distributors grew the National Aloe Science Council, Inc. (NASC), created in 1981 by concerned aloe vera businesspeople. This nonprofit association, based in Austin, Texas, represents many members of the aloe vera industry, encourages research, and creates a reliable source of information about the plant and the manufacturing of its products. Today the NASC includes growers, processors, manufacturers, and marketers who have adopted an industry code of ethics and have agreed to make no claims about aloe vera's health and beauty benefits without scientific research and technical data to support such claims.

However, like the plant it promotes, the NASC has become a point of controversy in the aloe vera community. Some members have withdrawn from the NASC because they found it ineffective in regulating the aloe vera industry. Disagreements over standards for evaluating and labeling the aloe vera content of products have created a major roadblock in the organization's campaign to set standards for the industry. Proposals for stronger regulations are being made by the FDA and the U.S. Department of Health and Human Services to establish a more aggressive tracking and regulating system in the industry as a means of further protecting consumers. Part of the problem lies in the fact that many companies are privately owned and are not required by law to provide or reveal financial records, resources, and other pertinent information that could be beneficial to consumers.

Claims about the effectiveness of aloe vera products are so voluminous and, for the most part, unsubstantiated that they appear more like myth than fact. But many aloe vera proponents believe that the plant has beneficial properties and is safe when used appropriately. Throughout the world, people have given aloe vera a permanent place in their medicine cabinets, incorporated it into their diets, and made a practice of using only aloe-containing cosmetics. For them, seeing and feeling the results of aloe vera is reason enough to believe.

A More Scientific Approach

Today, more than ever, aloe is moving in a new direction that demands the respect and interest of scientists around the world. The applications of aloe are being more clearly defined as researchers begin to identify and recommend new treatments that use aloe vera both in its natural state as a topical ointment and in an injectable form.

Research is being conducted by Dr. Wendell Winters, president of the Aloe Research Foundation, associate professor of Microbiology at the University of Texas Health Science Center at San Antonio, and world-recognized expert in aloe bioactivity. What makes his work significant is that other scientists have evaluated and critically reviewed it, and continue to do so.

"The research we're doing today on aloe substances we have identified gives academic credibility to those aloe components in products being sold commercially if active aloe is actually being used in those products," says Dr. Winters. "As scientists who have dedicated much of our lives to aloe research, our focus is more in tune with eastern philosophy where the medicine (or aloe) is most effective when taken in low doses over a long period of time, rather than the high dose, quick fix, cure-all approach that many salespeople try to push with aloe products today," he adds.

A LIVING
LEGEND 2

It is difficult to accurately trace the history of aloe vera. The plant is said to have originated in southern Africa and to have been taken across trade routes into other warm climates in Europe, Spain, East India, China, the West Indies, South America, and other parts of the western hemisphere. As aloe vera spread throughout the world so did romantic legends and folklore about its uses.

Images of the aloe vera plant have been found carved on Egyptian walls and coffins from 4000 B.C. It's believed that the Egyptians valued the plant most for its use as a drug but that it was also brought as a gift to the pharaohs' funerals. The translucent gel inside the leaves is said to have been a secret beauty treatment of Egyptian queens Cleopatra and Nefertiti.

The smooth complexions of the Mayan Indian women of the Yucatan are also attributed to the use of the gel. North and Central American Indians have long relied on aloe vera gel to treat burns and prevent blisters. And myth has it that Florida's

Seminole Indians described the fountain of youth as water that flowed from the center of a cluster of aloe vera plants.

Aloe vera has long been considered to bring good fortune and repel evil. Hundreds of years ago, Africans hung clumps of aloe vera above their doorways to ward off evil spirits. Today, Egyptians hang aloe vera plants over the doorways of new homes as a symbol of hope and good fortune to those who live there.

In Mexico, potted aloe vera plants are placed near the front doors of houses so that people who walk through will have good intentions, and "Mexican businessmen hang aloe vera above the entrances to their stores so that people who walk in will bring good business," according to Juan Chavira, Ph.D., J.D.

"In some countries, friends wrap an aloe vera plant in paper and give it to newlyweds without planting or watering it," says Bill McAnalley, Ph.D., former vice president and research director of Carrington Laboratories in Dallas, Texas. "As long as the plant continues to put out new shoots, the couple is supposed to have good luck."

According to McAnalley, when aloe vera is uprooted, the large outer leaves die and the water from those leaves travels to the center of the plant to make new leaves. "Most plants will shrivel up after a few days without water, but aloe vera continues to put out new shoots for up to seven years without water," he says.

THE DISCOVERY OF ALOE VERA'S HEALING POWERS

The first recorded pharmaceutical use of aloe was found on Sumerian clay tablets from 1750 B.C. The plant was also mentioned in the *Papyrus Ebers*—an Egyptian medical treatise—as well as in the *Egyptian Book of Remedies,* both written in approximately 1550 B.C. In the sixth century B.C., Arab traders introduced the use of aloe vera as a laxative to other parts of the world, including Persia, India, Tibet, and Malaysia.

The Greek philosopher Aristotle wrote about the beneficial medicinal effects of aloe vera. Historians believe it was Aristotle, tutor of Alexander the Great, who persuaded the king to conquer the island of Socotra, off the east African coast, for its large aloe vera crop.

"Alexander the Great's troops reportedly uprooted the plants and took them into battle to treat wounded soldiers. When someone got hurt, they'd take a leaf from a plant and wrap it around the wound to help it heal," says McAnalley. "They valued the plant's ability to survive unplanted because it sometimes took months, even years, before the plants reached the front lines."

References to aloe are also found throughout the Bible. It was brought as a gift to honor the birth of Jesus, and the Book of John (19:39), in the New Testament, states that Jesus' body was anointed with a mixture of aloes and myrrh according to Jewish burial customs.

In the first century A.D., Dioscorides, a Roman physician, and Pliny the Elder, author of *Historia Naturalis,* both wrote of using aloe extracts to treat wounds, stomach aches, constipation, headaches, insect bites, hair loss, mouth and gum diseases, kidney ailments, and skin irritations.

Explorers Marco Polo and Christopher Columbus also wrote of using aloe vera as a curative. The Spanish Jesuit priests of the sixteenth and seventeenth centuries, known to be scholars and physicians, are credited with having brought the plant with them from Spain and Portugal when they accompanied explorers to the New World.

According to the *United States Dispensatory and Physician's Pharmacology,* aloe vera was used in North America to heal wounds and burns during the sixteenth and seventeenth centuries.

The use of aloe vera was limited during the last half of the seventeenth century, when European scholars failed to verify the pharmacological value of aloe vera except for its cathartic action. Some believe that the researchers' findings were probably based on the fact that they did not use fresh gel. This, combined with the twentieth-century development of synthetic drugs, could be the reason why interest in the plant waned until the 1930s and 1940s, when it was used to treat radiation burns, and again in the late 1960s, when methods for stabilizing aloe vera products were developed.

MODERN USES OF ALOE

Modern medical research on aloe vera began in 1935, when C. E. Collins, M.D., and his son Creston followed the lead of the Seminole Indians and began treating burns, caused by the unsophisticated X-ray techniques of the time, with aloe vera. They discovered that the wounds healed more quickly and left less scar tissue when fresh aloe vera gel was applied than when other treatments were used.

In 1937 and 1939, J. E. Crew, M.D., used fresh aloe leaves and later pharmaceutical aloe vera ointments to treat eczema, skin ulcers, thermal burns, and sunburn. He found that aloe vera worked to reduce pain, itching, and scarring and to fight infection.

Medical researchers who followed up the studies conducted

by Collins and Crew to identify the healing effects of aloe vera gave the active principles of the plant such names as the "wound-healing hormone" and "biogenic stimulator."

The first extensive clinical tests using aloe vera to treat third-degree radiation burns on white rats were conducted by Professor Tom Rowe of the Medical College of Virginia. Rowe used various preparations of aloe vera, including fresh gel, partially decomposed gel, fresh rind, extracts of dried rind, and an ointment made from dried aloe vera. His studies showed that regardless of the condition of the leaves of the plant, aloe vera was effective. Rowe also discovered that although the healing agent in aloe vera is concentrated in the rind, it is also present in the gel. Finally, Rowe discovered that the ointments prepared from the leaves were not effective. This was because the variable nature of the juice inside the leaves makes it difficult to stabilize and use in a commercial preparation.

Because of the inconclusive findings, interest in using aloe vera for radiation burns and other skin conditions dwindled until 1959, when the Atomic Energy Commission (now the Nuclear Regulatory Commission) funded a study to produce an aloe vera ointment and test its effectiveness in treating radiation burns. The test results showed that aloe vera speeded up the healing time of ulcers caused by X-rays and reduced the formation of scar tissue. Since then, similar results in treating serious burns and leg ulcers have been shown in studies conducted in the United States and other countries.

Even so, no one had perfected a method for stabilizing the aloe vera gel. After a few days at room temperature the gel in the ointment began to decompose and lose its chemical effectiveness. The inability to stabilize aloe vera and the development of improved X-ray techniques, together with new methods for treating diseases once treated by X-rays, contributed to a decline in the use of aloe vera.

During the late 1960s, however, interest in aloe vera once more surged as methods for concentrating and stabilizing aloe vera gel were discovered. Stabilization prevents deterioration of the plant's chemical activity, extending its shelf life and its effectiveness. Several companies selling aloe vera products take credit for developing the first stabilization process, and each company claims that its process produces superior products.

Today, aloe vera juices, skin and hair care products, and pharmaceutical creams for treating burns and other injuries are the basis for a burgeoning industry in this country and others. Aloe vera is used by skin and hair care specialists, physicians, dentists, ophthalmologists, and veterinarians in the United States, Japan, Germany, the Soviet Union, and other countries.

According to the NASC, more than a thousand papers on the uses and effectiveness of aloe vera have been published by research scientists. These scientists are discovering that while one plant couldn't possibly be a cure-all for everything from acne to venereal disease, aloe vera does have certain beneficial qualities that need further investigation.

BOTANICALS—
A NATURAL PART OF MEDICINE

Today many physicians have discovered the value of aloe vera products to treat many health conditions. Using a plant-based product should not seem surprising, since many of the drugs we know today are based on plant derivatives or are patterned after substances found in plants.

According to Norman R. Farnsworth, Ph.D., (research professor of pharmacognosy at the College of Pharmacy, University of Illinois at Chicago), a survey carried out in 1981 showed that over the previous twenty-five years, 50 percent of all prescriptions dispensed from community pharmacies in the United States, including antibiotics and antifungal products, had an active ingredient obtained from a plant source. He reports that "in 1980, the American public paid eight billion dollars for those prescriptions and another half-a-billion dollars for plant-containing over-the-counter drugs."

Professor Winters, of the University of Texas Health Science Center at San Antonio, believes that aloe is truly a "pharmacy in a plant" because of its numerous healing abilities.

"There is a wide range of aloe components that have been widely recognized and investigated that have definite pharmacologic-like effects, thus generally confirming the folk medicine uses of aloe vera which are and can be truly valuable to us," he says.

Dr. Winters believes that the significant findings he and his co-workers have uncovered about the nature of the aloe components will permit further identification and rigorous analysis of them. The response stimulated by aloe substances in the immune system may bring us closer to a cure for current and emerging infectious diseases. The focus of the scientific world has been on the identification of immune-active ingredients and responses to aloe purified substances. Aloe has mostly been used topically, but more work is being done to determine its effectiveness internally and for treatment of ulcers and deep wounds that usually must heal from the inside out.

Although a similar analysis has not been performed in other

countries, Farnsworth says that the World Health Organization estimates that 65 percent of the 4.5 billion people in the world use plant-derivative drugs as a primary source of treatment.

There are more than 120 drugs made today that are based on plants, according to Farnsworth. "Morphine and codeine come from opium poppies, the ulcer drug atropine comes from a species of *Duboisia,* and a high blood pressure medication, reserpine, is a derivative from the Indian plant *Rauwolfia.* The heart medication digitalis contains about thirty plant substances and the birth control pill is indirectly derived from a Mexican yam."

Although many of the active ingredients (the chemical constituents that lead to certain effects) of plants can be reproduced in the laboratory, drug companies continue to make pharmaceuticals with plant extracts. "Plant material is believed to cause less side effects than synthetic drugs," says Farnsworth.

It is a plant's active ingredient that drug companies work to identify, extract, and patent in order to create a new drug. According to Farnsworth, most aloe vera companies manufacture products using the crude extracts of the plant, so they cannot patent their products or earn an exclusive right to market aloe vera products. Some companies are conducting studies to identify the active ingredient or ingredients in aloe vera and are working to design a drug patterned after the ingredient(s) so that they can patent the drug for exclusive production.

The future of aloe vera, then, may include not only products made from the natural gel and juice but new drugs patterned after this special plant.

THE INSIDE STORY: HOW ALOE VERA WORKS 3

How has a plant whose use dates back thousands of years survived the competition of modern medicine in treating a variety of health conditions? Why are people investing millions of dollars to identify the specific properties of aloe vera? What is it about this unusual plant that makes it a valuable cosmetic and pharmaceutical ingredient?

With all the attention aloe vera has received, even people who are skeptical about the claims made for it wonder whether there is some truth in what they hear. The confirmed aloe vera users are curious because they want to learn as much as possible about how the plant affects the body to produce the results they have witnessed.

Physicians, scientists, and aloe vera product manufacturers are working to unlock the mysteries behind the biochemical makeup of the plant. The more we can learn about aloe vera, the easier it will be to identify the active ingredients in it, understand how they affect the body, and formulate products that will yield maximum benefits. This research will also make it possible to replicate the active ingredients in aloe vera and produce synthetic drugs to achieve the same results.

To understand how aloe vera works, it's important to realize that aloe vera has two main constituents: the aloe drug and the aloe gel. The aloe drug is derived from the juice obtained from cells beneath the tough outer skin of the plant. When dried and purified, the aloe drug yields extracts that contain resins, anthraquinones, and anthraglycosides. The crystallized anthraglycosides in the aloe extracts are called aloin, a yellow substance with an extremely bitter taste that has been used for centuries as a laxative. The main ingredient of aloin is an anthraquinone glycoside called barbaloin, known pharmaceutically as aloe-emodin.

When taken internally, aloin has a strong cathartic effect, so it is often combined with other ingredients to produce a milder laxative. In addition to its laxative properties, the aloe drug has sunscreening properties and is often used in cosmetics to protect the skin from harsh ultraviolet rays.

Early in the twentieth century, when the FDA began requiring chemical analyses before recognizing new drugs, aloin was the only chemical in aloe vera that could properly be identified and analyzed. Therefore, aloin became the only part of the aloe vera plant accepted for medical use by the FDA. Other uses of aloe vera were relegated to the classification of folk remedies. In the last twenty years, however, since the stabilization process for aloe vera gel was developed, scientists have made in-depth studies of aloe vera gel and the juices derived from it. This research has created new interest in its properties and how it affects the human body, both taken internally and used externally.

ALOE GEL: A STOREHOUSE OF NUTRIENTS

The aloe vera plant has developed many special characteristics to survive in extremely dry climates and endure weeks, even years, without moisture. Root systems supply the majority of plant species with the nutrients that they need to survive from the soil. The root system of the aloe vera plant, however, is not the primary mechanism for food and water storage. Instead, the gel inside the leaves of an aloe vera plant is its lifeblood, rich in nutrition and moisture.

"Aloe vera seems more like an animal in terms of its ability to survive," says Clinton Howard, founder of Carrington Laboratories. "The plant can be uprooted and live for years on its internal supply of water, chemicals, and enzymes. And it's the special chemical make-up that gives aloe vera a wider range of healing characteristics than any other plant."

Part of the healing properties of aloe vera can be attributed to its high water content. The gel found inside the soft, pulpy leaves contains approximately 96 percent water. When aloe vera is used on human tissue, the water is carried to the injured area without closing off the air necessary to repair tissue.

In addition to water, aloe vera gel consists of hundreds of different substances. Studies performed at the University of Chicago by Martin C. Robson, M.D., John P. Heggers, Ph.D., and William Hagstrom, Jr., M.D., showed that aloe vera includes inorganic substances such as sodium, potassium, chloride, calcium, and phosphorus. Organic compounds that were found include glucose, protein, cholesterol, triglycerides, salicylic acid, and traces of magnesium and zinc.

The protein in aloe vera contains eighteen of the twenty amino acids found in the body. The quantity of amino acids is believed to be too small for aloe vera to be considered as a food supplement, but it's generally agreed that the amino acids do help build healthy skin.

Reports of the nutritional content of aloe vera vary tremendously. Like other vegetable juices, stabilized aloe vera juice is said to be rich in vitamins, including vitamins A, B_1, B_2, B_3, B_6, C, and E. While some of these vitamins are found naturally in the plant, others are added during the stabilization process.

Forever Living Products, a multi-level marketing company based in Phoenix, Arizona, also contends that aloe vera contains vitamin B_{12} in small amounts. In a company brochure, Arnold Fox, M.D., an internist and cardiologist, and director and medical consultant of the American Institute of Health and Stress Management of Beverly Hills, reported that the aloe vera juice he tested contained an average of 50 picograms of B_{12} per milliliter. (In the average person, the blood levels of vitamin B_{12} are said to range from 200 to 1,100 picograms per milliliter.) Other people in the aloe vera industry, however, say that there has not been enough research conducted to substantiate such claims.

There is also some disagreement about the source of the anthraquinones found in aloe vera. While some believe the anthraquinones are only found in the latex, others say that they are also present in trace amounts in the gel, contributing to its anti-inflammatory and pain-killing properties.

Bill Wolfe, D.D.S., a dentist in Albuquerque, New Mexico, uses aloe vera gel products to help reduce swelling and pain after oral surgery and other dental procedures. According to Wolfe, anthraquinones occur naturally in nature, much like endorphins (the body's natural morphine, which is released from the brain when we laugh or exercise for a prolonged period of time and which became well known through Norman Cousins's book *Anatomy Of An Illness*). "The anthraquinones in aloe vera have an anesthetic effect, meaning that the aloe plant numbs while it heals," says Dr. Wolfe.

Aloe vera gel has several distinct healing properties. It has the ability to kill certain bacteria, fungi, and viruses. It also has the ability to dilate capillaries, which increases the blood supply in the area to which it is applied. When applied to injured tissue, the gel penetrates and anesthetizes tissue, relieving pain and itching. Aloe vera's anti-inflammatory properties reduce swelling of the skin and muscles.

Sheldon Saul Hendler, M.D., Ph.D., an internal medicine specialist in San Diego, California, and author of *The Complete Guide to Anti-Aging Nutrients* (Simon and Schuster), says that anti-inflammatory substances in aloe vera could account for some of its benefits in accelerating the healing of mild burns and other skin irritations: "It may work as a topical ointment for mild burns and mosquito bites, but don't look for miraculous results."

One of the most valuable roles aloe vera plays in maintaining healthy skin or helping wounded skin to heal is serving as a transport mechanism to carry other substances into the layers of the skin. "Picture aloe vera as a pick-up truck," says Elizabeth Burdick, M.S., a biochemist and skin therapist who is co-owner of Dermatheray, Inc., in Encinitas, California. "When combined with other skin care ingredients, aloe loads the water, amino acids, vitamins, minerals, and nutrients present in those substances into the truck and transports them into the dermal layer of the skin."

Exactly how aloe gel works externally in healing wounds or maintaining healthy skin has not yet been proved. But Burdick says there are two main theories. "One is that when applied to the skin the chemical properties of aloe vera increase cell regeneration at a very rapid rate. The other theory is that the extract contains enzymes that effect chemical changes, which in turn intensify healing."

Laboratory tests to determine whether aloe vera increases cell replacement were performed by Wendell Winters, Ph.D., at the University of Texas Health Science Center in San Antonio. Dr. Winters applied fresh aloe vera extracts to cultured human cells that had been "wounded" to resemble cut skin. The study showed that treatment with fresh aloe vera juice increased the healing process and the growth of new cells. When processed aloe vera extracts were similarly tested, Dr. Winters found that some inhibited the growth or killed cultured cells. "We have now isolated a complex of growth factors and are in the process of completing testing in human and animal situations which will mean a reevaluation of aloe vera with more scientific support." It is encouraging that support has been found within scientific research studies being done in laboratories around the world as scientists like Dr. Winters move toward a better understanding of the immune-activating ingredients found in aloe.

Carrington Laboratories reproduced Dr. Winter's study. "We grew human skin cells and found that aloe vera does speed up the growth of human cells by stimulating the fibroblasts, which are the healing cells in the skin," says McAnalley. "But we also discovered that the laxative drug in aloe vera kills healthy cells.

"Pluses and minuses are expected in any natural medicine," McAnalley continues. "The presence of yellow sap in aloe vera juices and gels kills cells at any dilution. We caution people against using the leaves from aloe vera plants to treat burns. Instead, we suggest that they use aloe vera creams and juices that have been made through special techniques designed to reduce the sap to an insignificant level."

But many people make a regular practice of using fresh aloe vera to treat skin irritations, cuts, and burns and have found no adverse effects. Rachel Perry, owner of Rachel Perry Natural Cosmetics, based in Chatsworth, California, and author of *Reverse the Aging Process of Your Face,* not only uses aloe vera in her products but uses the fresh gel directly from the leaf for minor first aid. "If I get burned, bruised, or have swollen skin tissue, I cut open an aloe vera leaf and place the leaf, gel side down, directly on the irritation," says Perry. "If the gel dries and the pain or swelling has not subsided, I cut a second leaf and repeat the process."

Dr. Wolfe believes that fresh aloe vera is effective, but that using commercial aloe vera products is more practical. "You can't carry a leaf around in your purse or take it to the office," he says. "Since the aloe vera raw gel is mostly water, commercial products are often more potent than the plant itself because they have higher concentrations of aloe gel and its active ingredients. Plus, commercial products have a longer shelf life than the raw gel."

Bill Coats, R.Ph., and Spanky Stephens, co-authors of *Healing Winners: Treating Athletic Injuries with Aloe Vera,* say that, although the chemical reason is not yet understood, using fresh aloe vera works best when the gel is left inside the leaf after the leaf is split, and not as well when the gel is used alone or in a gel-soaked bandage. They do agree, though, that using gel directly from the plant presents limitations. They say that because aloe vera grows best in hot, dry, arid climates, the plant does not survive in most areas of the United States. In addition, when large quantities are needed, using fresh plants or refrigerated fresh gel is unrealistic.

IDENTIFYING ALOE'S ACTIVE INGREDIENT

Although scientists have identified much of the biochemistry of aloe vera, further research is aimed at determining the exact way those components work together to heal the body.

The complex chemical make-up of aloe vera makes it difficult to break down, even with all the modern instrumentation, but aloe experts believe that aloe triggers the healing mechanism in the body, whether the problem is an ulcer, a burn, acne, or some other type of cellular damage. But whatever is in aloe vera that makes it function is in very minute quantities. In their own ways, time, and financial abilities, people interested in aloe vera are trying to identify the trigger mechanism in aloe vera that sets off a specific response in the body, causing a healing reaction to take place.

Bill Coats believes that it is the synergy—the joint action—among the ingredients in aloe vera that makes it effective in treating a variety of health conditions. "The amount of amino acids, vitamins, enzymes, anthraquinone complexes, and other components in aloe vera is very small, and [they] will not work by themselves to produce desired results," says Coats, "but when they work together, they help to heal the body. You can find one ingredient that kills bacteria and another that kills fungus, but I don't believe there is only one component that is responsible for the majority of health claims made about aloe vera.

Clinton Howard, founder of Carrington Laboratories, says his company is betting millions of dollars that it has identified the active ingredient in aloe vera that promotes healing. "It has taken us several years and an investment of $9 million in laboratory research, to isolate the active ingredient in aloe vera and determine how it acts," says Howard. "We will then use this research to develop what will be a new family of drugs patterned after the active ingredients."

In double-blind studies evaluating aloe vera's effectiveness in treating ulcers, Carrington Laboratories tested a drug it extracted from aloe vera against the control Cimetidine, one of the major ulcer drugs. The lab reported that it had never seen a drug give the kind of protection that aloe vera gave.

"Aloe vera definitely had a healing effect on ulcers, and it heals in a way that is entirely different than other ulcer medications on the market," says Howard. "Most of the current ulcer drugs on the market work by reducing the production of hydrochloric acid in the stomach. Ours may have a surface action effect, and coat the stomach in much the same way as the drugs Mylanta and Maalox."

McAnalley explains that Carrington Laboratories does not really know how the new aloe-patterned drug works. "That is a common phenomenon with drugs," he explains. "No one really knows how aspirin works; we just know that it does. We used to think that aspirin worked on headache receptors, but now we think it works on prostaglandin synthesis. We don't know whether this new ulcer drug makes the natural coating in the stomach work better or if it serves as a partial coating itself."

Carrington Laboratories contracted with a research group to conduct human clinical studies using the aloe vera–derived drug Carrington developed, called Carrysin, in the treatment of ulcers. At the same time, continued research in their own lab indicated that the aloe vera–derived drug worked as an immune stimulant. "The active ingredient in aloe vera stimulates our body's macrophage, one of the white blood cells that controls the immune system," says Howard. "We also discovered that Carrysin causes macrophage to put out increased amounts of prostaglandin, an anti-inflammatory product."

With this discovery coming in the midst of the AIDS crisis, Carrington Laboratories decided to forego the research on aloe's use in ulcer drugs and instead develop it to treat diseases for which there are no products on the market. "There's no sense competing with a half dozen ulcer drugs on the market, when we could develop a drug to treat AIDS, for which there is no safe, approved treatment," says Howard. "We have concentrated our research in the areas of AIDS, colitis, and bedsores."

Carrington Laboratories has also shown that in double-blind studies, Carrysin reduces the infectivity of certain viruses, such as Herpes I and Herpes II, in human cells.

New methods for evaluating the active ingredient in aloe vera are covered by patents. Carrington Laboratories has filed patent applications in 37 countries, and patent claims in the United States have been allowed.

Carrington Laboratories is not alone in its quest to derive the most benefits, both therapeutic and financial, from aloe vera. Dentist Bill Wolfe, D.D.S., of Albuquerque, has been working for the last four years with Eugene Zimmermann, M.A., D.D.S., professor of pathology at Baylor College of Dentistry in Dallas, Texas, to identify the potential of using aloe vera gel in dentistry. "I was excited about the results I was seeing from using aloe vera in my practice," says Dr. Wolfe. "It seemed to have bactericidal effects on dental plaque and helped to stimulate healing after surgery, but I wanted to prove its effectiveness and safeness scientifically. Today we have produced an aloe-based oral gel used by dentists for its bactericidal, virucidal, and anti-inflammatory effects, and a toothpaste which will not only clean teeth but help heal the gums as well.

Dr. Wolfe goes on to say "aloe vera has been around for thousands of years, but it is just coming to the forefront of medicine and dentistry. The benefits people derive from aloe vera are proof of what it can do."

THE MAKING OF
ALOE VERA 4

As a houseplant, aloe vera needs minimal care and attention. Grown for commercial use, however, the plant cannot merely be left to the custody of nature. Aloe vera, though hardy, has a few natural enemies and must be shielded against frost, gophers, and wind.

The Rio Grande Valley of South Texas—with its rich mixture of clay, silt, and sandy soil, warm, humid weather, and efficient irrigation systems—is the primary producer of aloe in the United States, although it is also grown in central and southern Florida. Outside this country, the plant grows in the semitropical regions of Mexico, South Africa, Australia, Jamaica, Curaçao, Aruba, Bonaire, Venezuela, and the Caribbean.

Aloe farmers say they have even shipped plants to Korea to be grown in hothouses. The government of Taiwan has also shown interest in growing aloe.

The Terry Corporation, an aloe vera processor and private label manufacturer in Melbourne, Florida, has been growing aloe vera plants hydroponically (in a nutrient solution). "Hydroponics has been a successful method of growing crops for many years," explains the company's president Vernon Pruitt. "The method is now being applied to aloe vera. Although the results appear promising, it is really too early to tell how well this type of growing will work in the long run. While a healthy plant is certainly produced, the efficacy of such a plant has not been fully determined. In addition, the cost of hydroponic growing is still too high for the grower to compete with more conventional methods."

In the field, aloe vera plants are placed in rows divided by irrigation ditches, which provide space for mechanical cultivation. Before planting, the soil is gently turned over and fertilized. Depending on the size of the starter plants, an aloe vera field should yield a large crop the first year and continue to produce a large crop for five to ten years.

Growing aloe is a labor-intensive business. Plants must be planted, cultivated, and harvested by hand. That, along with the processing required, is why Aloe Laboratories of Texas, Inc., estimates that an established aloe vera crop will sell for approximately ten cents a pound. (The average yield per acre per year is between 100,000 and 120,000 pounds.)

A gallon of aloe vera juice sells for between $4.50 and $6.50 wholesale. The retail price jumps significantly because of the middlemen involved between the aloe vera farms and the store shelf. A gallon of aloe vera juice in a health food store sells for between $12 and $20 a gallon; some multi-level marketing companies get up to $27 a gallon for their aloe vera juice.

Great care is taken to produce healthy aloe vera plants with thick, green leaves that will yield a maximum quantity of juice.

Typically, aloes are mostly pest resistant, as the acrid lemon-colored sap in the leaves wards off insects, animals, and birds. Most aloe growers avoid using chemical pesticides and herbicides, and some let geese into the fields to eat insects that are uncovered by plowing.

One thing most growers don't worry much about is the reproduction of aloe vera plants. Aloe vera is a continuous crop and propagates very rapidly. While seeds from the aloe vera flower are responsible for some propagation, most new plants grow off the root of a "mother" plant. Within eight to nine months the aloe vera "pups" are nearly as large as the "mother" and are replanted in open fields. Most farmers wait to harvest aloe vera plants until they are at least fourteen to eighteen months old because mature plants have a 60 percent yield based on the weight of the gel, whereas immature plants have only a 30 percent yield.

The aloe vera leaves are generally ready for processing when they weigh one and a half pounds or more, measure about twenty-four inches long and four to six inches across at the bottom of the leaf, and are from one to one and a half inches thick. They are cut off near the base of the plant at a point that is high enough to keep the immature inner leaves intact. Typically, only two or three leaves are removed at a time, leaving eight to twelve remaining on the plant.

Once aloe vera is harvested, it is processed almost immediately: "We try to process the leaves on the same day they're picked, but sometimes we'll have some left over and those won't be processed until the next day," says Smith about his own company. "During the summer, leaves have to be processed the same day, but in the cooler months we can wait a day or even refrigerate the leaves over a weekend."

When the leaves are grown by one company and sold to another for processing, they are often shipped cross-country in refrigerator trucks. Each leaf is individually wrapped to prevent any damage that could cause the gel to drain out or the yellow sap to mix with the gel.

Many firms that sell aloe vera products are also involved in growing and processing the plant as well as manufacturing the products in their own facilities. Aloe Laboratories of Texas in Harlingen has several operations: "We have 200 acres on which we grow our own aloe," says Ray Henry. "We sell some plants to nurseries and sell aloe vera leaves as a crop to competitors. We also process the gel from the leaves into a finished product to be used as a raw material, which we then sell worldwide. Additionally, we manufacture our own product line of cosmetics and produce private label cosmetics for companies around the world."

Other companies that grow aloe vera manufacture and sell products under their own labels and also sell processed gel to other "private label" companies.

Farmers and manufacturers often employ innovative ways to ship their products overseas. Because of the high cost of freight, they often freeze-dry aloe vera, which can be reconstituted to make a drink or cosmetic when it reaches the destination. The freeze-dried aloe vera is cheaper to ship and easier to use than liquid aloe vera in the preparation of some products. But though there is no evidence, it is thought by some that the liquid aloe vera does a better job than the freeze-dried.

PROCESSING ALOE VERA

The most precious commodity of the aloe vera plant is the juice, made from the clear gel stored inside the leaf. Considered "liquid gold" by the multimillion dollar aloe vera industry, the gel is usually removed from the leaves with painstaking care to insure that the yellow sap–containing tubules that lie beneath the skin are not punctured.

"It's impossible to obtain aloe vera without breaking through the rind," says Clinton Howard, founder of Carrington Laboratories. "We have two processes to reduce contamination. One is in the way we hand fillet the leaves and the other is a process to remove any sap that finds its way into the gel."

Howard reminds the consumers that a drink that contains the yellow sap is also a laxative: "The laxative in aloe vera is a drug laxative. Most gastroenterologists will say that you should not use drug laxatives on a daily basis," continues Howard, "because they are gastric irritants which can poison the enzyme system in the lining of the stomach. Drinking aloe vera with a content of yellow sap above ten parts per million is not a good idea."

After the leaves are harvested, they are washed and the tips and bottoms are removed. The leaves are then sliced open in a way that is similar to how a fish is filleted, and the outside rind is removed, exposing the gel inside. While many aloe vera manufacturers rely on machines to fillet the leaves, others believe that hand filleting produces the cleanest gel.

In the automated method, the leaves are processed through a machine that mechanically scrapes the inner leaf. "The blade of the machine is set so that, for the most part, the tubules in the rind are not ruptured," says Don Smothers. "But to do that, some of the gel must be left in the leaf." Whether the leaves are machine or hand processed, some 50 percent of the leaf is discarded as waste product.

When the leaves are filleted by hand, the workers use knives to cut away the outer rind—including the layer containing the latex—and then scoop out gel. High labor costs, however, make this method expensive.

McAnalley, who prefers hand-filleted aloe vera, says that the imperfections of a leaf are often not apparent until it has been skinned. He believes that once the leaves are put into a machine for filleting there is little quality control. "A machine can't discern a good leaf from a bad one and doesn't see bad spots, like those caused from frost damage, which may mean that yellow sap has invaded the gel," asserts McAnalley. "It would be like picking potatoes and not cutting out the bad spots. If all the leaves were good, you wouldn't have a problem."

McAnalley adds that one of the big frustrations with machine filleting is the variable leaf size. "You get the machine adjusted to one size and bigger leaves come through, and the machine starts to put a lot of yellow sap out," he observes.

"It's cheaper to machine fillet," McAnalley says, "because a machine can do the work of fifty or sixty people, and it doesn't get sick and isn't paid overtime. We think hand filleting results in a better product, but we're sure that with new technology a machine will be made that will deliver the type of product we want."

After the leaves are filleted, the inner jelly-like pulp is ground by a blender. The aloe is then reduced to a near-liquid state. Fresh aloe degrades when exposed to air, so the gel must be treated to prevent oxidation and loss of the plant's vitamins, minerals, amino acids, and other ingredients. Most companies stabilize the gel by pasteurization and the addition of preservatives, but processing techniques vary from company to company. "Just as the preservative sodium benzoate is added to soft drinks to keep bacteria from growing, we add preservatives to processed aloe vera," explains McAnalley.

While some firms advertise that their products contain no preservatives and are not pasteurized, most agree that aloe vera, like any other vegetable, must be preserved once it's been processed, unless it's kept refrigerated or vacuum sealed in a can.

McAnalley says that some companies originally claimed that their products killed bacteria. "We took fresh aloe vera and added it to the same organism that one company claimed their product could kill, and it didn't do anything," he says. "We've had that confirmed by independent microbiologists. We think it was the preservatives added to that product which might have killed the microorganisms, not the aloe vera," he continues. "Just as it's the sodium benzoate in Coke which keeps the bacteria from growing, not the Coke itself."

Bacterial growth in aloe vera products can be controlled by pasteurization. The product is brought up to a high temperature—165 degrees Fahrenheit for thirty minutes—then mixed with preservatives. Pasteurization will kill all the bacteria that are present at the time, and the chemical preservatives will prevent bacteria from growing after bottling. Pasteurization isn't necessary, but many manufacturers think it's the best method when used along with preservatives.

Not everyone agrees that the heating process is advantageous. "Almost everybody heats their product to sterilize it, but I feel if you can keep from doing that you'll have a better product," Don Smothers explains. "Heating destroys many enzymes and changes a lot of the protein structures of the product. We use a fugitive sterilizing agent. This is an agent that sterilizes the product without entering any chemical reaction with the aloe vera, and the agent is then completely removed, all without the necessity of any heat."

After stabilization, the processed aloe gel may be filtered to remove the pulp, depending on the type of product the company makes. For cosmetics and some juice drinks the filtered aloe is preferred, but some people like unfiltered drinks because they say the pulp is a good source of fiber. According to Henry, "None of our testing has shown any benefit to leaving the pulp in, and most of our customers prefer a juice that is free of pulp."

Carrington Laboratories, on the other hand, believes that when you remove the pulp, you remove a lot of what's good in the aloe vera plant. According to Howard, some manufacturers remove the pulp from the aloe vera gel and sell it to other companies. They then thicken the filtrated product by adding Irish moss extractive, known generically as carrageenin, to make it appear that the product hasn't been filtered. "In our view carrageenin should never be included in an aloe vera drink because studies have shown that it causes tumors in primates," says Howard.

In freeze-drying, the aloe vera gel is reduced to a powder. According to Smothers, most manufacturers use an additive, such as gum or resin, to form a matrix upon which the gel can agglomerate. "This makes it easier to reduce the material to a fine powder," he says, "but some processors claim to prepare the powdered aloe vera without any matrix."

Since keeping the gel free of hair and dirt is important during the processing, employees in aloe vera factories are sanitarily garbed in white lab coats, caps, and gloves. Quality control is typically high, and the products are tested for various properties such as color, viscosity, and pH balance.

ALOE'S NATURAL ENEMIES

There may be several ways to kill the bacteria that attack fresh aloe vera, but there is one threat to the plant that is not so easily controlled: frost.

Christmas Eve 1983 brought little cheer to Texas aloe vera growers, as the temperature plummeted to the freezing mark and remained there for fifty hours. Mother Nature changed the plans of many people who saw aloe vera as a lucrative crop and got into it only to have the bottom fall out. Some farmers simply plowed the aloe vera under and started thinking about planting other crops.

Since that freeze and the freeze that came the next year, growers have had little time for recovery, and today there are fewer people growing aloe vera in Texas. But some new growers have sprung up in warmer climates, such as the Caribbean, Mexico, and Australia. According to McAnalley, freezing ruins the quality of the leaves, often without affecting how they look on the outside. "A freeze can cause the yellow sap to get into the gel," he explains. "This makes for poor-quality products when used in cosmetics and inadvertently puts a laxative effect into the juice."

ALOE VERA AS A HOUSEPLANT

Cold winter temperatures make it impossible to keep potted aloe vera plants outdoors in most areas of the United States. Nevertheless, the spiny succulent can be grown successfully indoors provided its special needs are met.

It is important not to crowd the aloe vera. The diameter of the container must be at least half the length of its leaves. For example, a plant with twelve-inch leaves needs a container at least six inches in diameter. A healthy plant will outgrow its container in a short time. Plastic or heavy terra-cotta pots are best.

Ideally, aloe vera prefers bright, filtered light with a southern or eastern exposure; indoor plants can be kept in a western window as well. This plant likes fresh air, so keep it on a windowsill if possible.

The soil should dry out between waterings. For this reason, it is important to plant it in rapid-draining soil. High humidity can be harmful to this otherwise hardy houseplant, and since the thick leaves store moisture for days, the most important tip in the home care of aloe vera plants is to avoid overwatering them. To test your soil, put some of it in a pot and pour water over it. If the water stands or is slow to drain, add pumice to the soil to improve drainage. A good blend is 50 percent pumice to the same amount of potting soil.

The best way to determine when to water your aloe vera plant is the knuckle test. Poke your finger into the soil up to the first knuckle. If it is dry to that point, water.

Feed your aloe vera plant monthly except in winter, when the plant rests. A low-nitrogen fertilizer is best, but be sure to follow the directions on the package.

Aloe vera can be grown from cuttings (pups) or seeds, but it takes much longer to grow from seeds. Start with cuttings from someone else's plant, or buy a small plant from a garden shop.

A healthy aloe vera plant will outgrow its container quickly, and you may need to transplant it to separate it. Pups grow around the mother plant and crowd the pot. You can either plant the pups separately or place the entire plant into a larger pot.

The pups send out their own roots and detach easily from the mother, so the plant seems to fall apart when you lift it from the pot. To remove pups, gently lift them out of the soil. If any roots are torn, let the pup dry for three or four days; if not, it can be placed directly in soil. Pups must have healthy roots to grow successfully.

Though most growers claim the aloe vera leaves should be about three feet long to be effective for healing, the leaves of the houseplant can be used at one foot. Growing the plant in a pot dwarfs it, so the leaves will not grow as large as they would if the plant were growing in the ground.

In addition to its utilitarian role as a first-aid plant, aloe vera has a fairer side. The striking yellow and red clusters of flowers with their long, bent stems make aloe vera a popular decoration and have earned it the nickname "Candelabra."

THE BLOSSOMING
ALOE VERA INDUSTRY

As Americans buy fewer processed foods and scrutinize product labels for chemical additives, "natural" foods and products receive a bigger share of the shopping dollar. What could be more "natural" than the gel or juice from a plant? Whether it's the belief that the cool gel of aloe vera is better for the skin than synthetic ingredients or that drinking the juice will promote good health, the public demands aloe vera, and in turn, cash registers ring.

There are many companies in the United States selling, manufacturing, or processing aloe vera products. According to C. Ray Henry, President of CRH International, Inc., a consulting firm specializing in aloe vera products and marketing in Texas, the total estimated annual sales for aloe vera companies in the United States is increasing annually despite a decrease in the number of producers brought about by the ever-strengthening FDA regulations and control.

The first aloe vera company in the United States—Collins

Chemical Company, established in 1934 by C. E. Collins, M.D.—conducted some of the early medical research on the plant and published the first medical report on the use of aloe vera for treating X-ray burns in March 1935, according to Bob White, former owner of the House of Aloe in Chicago. "In 1967 I bought out the Collins Chemical Company. Prior to this, in 1963, I purchased another aloe company, Tru-Aloe Products, from Henry McCarty, a retired chemist living in the Blue Ridge Mountains of northern Georgia. McCarty had established his company in 1937 and 1938 in Miami and had aloe plantations growing south of Miami before World War II."

White first learned about aloe vera while working in Louisiana as a roadbuilder for his family-owned company. "I developed early stages of skin cancer from being out in the sun so much," White recalls. "The Shell Oil Company was putting in pipelines on a road project, and I asked one of the workmen why he could stay out in the sun with no adverse effects and I couldn't. He said that he and the others on his crew had discovered aloe vera while working in the oil fields in the Middle East. I tried using aloe vera after I was out in the sun and it seemed to protect my skin. Years later I went into the aloe vera business and began importing plants from Mexico into the Rio Grande Valley."

White says that in the United States, people in the oil industry were the first to recognize the benefits of aloe vera. "H. L. Hunt had an aloe vera company known as H.L.H. Aloe Vera," says White, "but it went out of business when he died. The president of Kewanee Oil Company also grew aloe vera on his private island in the Caribbean. Wealthy oil people cruising on their yachts would stop off at the island to pick aloe vera leaves to treat their sunburns."

Today, not only aloe vera product manufacturers but manufacturers of other products have taken advantage of the plant's intriguing history and commercial lure. Marketing departments of major companies have redesigned product labels to include banners announcing the addition of aloe vera.

"Aloe vera has high public awareness and is perceived by the consumer as being effective for a variety of uses," says Smothers. "Some companies advertise that their products contain aloe vera when in reality the products don't include much of the plant at all. While there's been a proliferation of the word 'aloe vera' on product labels, there probably isn't any more aloe vera sold today than there was three years ago. As the old saying among aloe vera growers goes, 'There's an awful lot more aloe vera sold than grown.'"

The name "aloe vera" sells products. Several years ago chemist Frank N. Romano and perfumier Joseph R. Liszka opened Key West Aloe, an 800-square-foot aloe vera company in Key West, Florida, to sell fragrances and aloe vera–containing cosmetics for men and women. "The first day we sold thirty-six dollars worth of products; today we are doing over seven million dollars in sales annually, and aloe vera has become a product that can be bought and sold on the commodities exchange," says Romano. "We have more than 100 employees and three buildings—two in Key West and one in Florida City. When we started, no one knew what aloe vera was. Now we put an aloe vera product on the shelf and people grab it."

If there is a Cinderella in the aloe vera business, it's probably Burn-Off Corporation in Irving, Texas, which produces and distributes aloe vera–based burn relief and sunscreen products through retail stores. Steve Finley, former president of Burn-

Off, says he started the company six years ago with $100. In 1988 the company projects gross sales in the millions of dollars—and the product is just beginning to be known in areas of the country outside the Texas coast.

"We started with the least amount of capital and have had a more rapid rate of growth than almost any other aloe vera company," says Finley. "Today we have a forty-two-item line of suntan products, including Burn-Off SPF 16, The Green Stuff, and Moisturizing Gel."

Finley attributes his company's success in part to the unique formulation of his product. "We were probably the first company to use aloe vera for sunburn relief and sunburn protection and distribute [those products] in the stores—not through multilevel marketing, which is how most aloe vera products in this country are sold," Finley explains.

"When we first went into business, Americans bought Solarcaine for burn relief and that was it," says Finley. "There was no nationally marketed aloe vera sunburn relief product. We formulated a burn relief cream that inhibited the pain from sunburn and moisturized the skin. Our product includes the pain killer lidocaine hydrochloride and 80 percent aloe vera gel. When you mix those two ingredients together you get the very best sunburn relief; it quells sunburn pain and replenishes the skin with moisture."

Finley believes that the success of his products is due to consumer demand for aloe vera sunburn products: "Today, every major suntan lotion company in the world has an aloe vera sunburn relief product and an aloe vera moisturizing product, and we feel that we were the pioneers in the market."

FROM RETAIL STORES
TO MULTI-LEVEL MARKETING

Aloe vera products reach consumers in two ways: through retail stores, including health food stores, supermarkets, and drug stores, and through multi-level marketing via independent distributors.

Like other well-known multi-level marketing companies, some aloe vera companies do not sell their products through retail outlets but rely solely on recruiting people to become product distributors. The distributors buy products for themselves, sell products to customers, and sponsor other distributors. They are encouraged to talk about the benefits of the company's products and sales plan to neighbors, co-workers, relatives, and friends. When people show interest in the product, they are invited to attend a meeting designed to "sell" them on the products and the business opportunity to sell the products. Once new recruits join a sales team, they attend frequent workshops to learn how to build their businesses and to acquaint themselves with new products.

Spreading the word about aloe vera requires aggressive marketing tactics. Many independent distributors exude a religious-like fervor in touting the virtues of the plant, and most tell of personal benefits derived from using it.

As they recruit new people to join the sales team, distributors move up through the hierarchy. They earn commissions not only on the products they sell but also on those sold by the distributors they sponsor.

Many people believe that since no medical claims can be made for aloe vera, direct marketing is the best way to sell aloe vera products. The testimonials about what aloe vera has done for other people intrigue new customers. And it's the hope that they will derive the same benefits that prompts them to buy the products.

Many aloe vera distributors work in other careers full time and sell aloe vera products to supplement their incomes. On the average, distributors may make anywhere from thirty dollars to a couple of thousand dollars a week.

To demonstrate faith in their products, many multi-level marketing companies offer a money-back guarantee if customers are not satisfied with the products. However, direct sales are based on educating the consumer about aloe vera and its uses, and some customers prefer buying products this way.

MEETING FDA REGULATIONS

No matter what avenue they choose to sell their products, most aloe vera product manufacturers make no claims for their products. They warn salespeople not to make promises for aloe vera or recommendations on how to use it. According to Smothers, the industry's stand not to make claims about products was reinforced in 1982 when the NASC got word of a rumor that the FDA was very close to shutting down the aloe vera industry. "We believed that the FDA had a few misconceptions about aloe, so we decided to go to Washington and find out what the problem was," recalls Smothers. "We discovered that the only definition the FDA had for aloe vera was the aloin-containing portion which is used as a laxative. The confusion came when the FDA started hearing people talk about using aloe vera as a drug. We told them that although there is a drug in the plant, there is a difference between the aloin-containing yellow sap and the gel, which does not contain much, if any, aloin. We consider the gel a food with health benefits similar to other foods, such as prunes, cabbage, and rutabaga. That was a revelation to some people at the FDA, and they suggested we talk to their Foods Division," Smothers continues. "We spoke with the Foods Division who agreed that the product is a food and will be recognized as a GRAS (Generally Recognized As Safe) product as long as it isn't modified with a non-GRAS product. Any preservative we use has to be on the GRAS list."

Smothers said that the NASC's work with the FDA defused many of the FDA's concerns. "There had been a lot of quackery associated with the product because there were a lot of unsubstantiated statements being made about the medicinal benefits of aloe vera in an effort to sell products," he explains. "The NASC has adopted a strict code of ethics and members have to comply by not making claims for their products."

Today, aloe vera has only been approved by the FDA as a natural flavoring substance in food, but not as a food supplement or a drug. As a result, the aloe vera industry relies on files of testimonial letters to "prove" their products' benefits.

According to Emil Corwin, information officer with the FDA, there are no specific regulations regarding aloe vera, only those that are required of all products: legitimate, non-misleading labeling and no excessive or exaggerated claims. "Some manufacturers of certain products try to get around this regulation for the label by placing brochures making these claims in the store where the product is sold," says Corwin. "There has been some litigation in cases where people have violated this regulation by using advertising as labeling."

To further protect consumers, the government is moving forward to pass even more stringent labeling laws. Beginning in

1995, the FDA requires specific information relative to food and substance values of each ingredient to be clearly identified on product labels. Part of the reason for this aggressive labeling move is that the FDA is concerned about exaggerated and unsubstantiated claims that lead consumers to believe that aloe vera products can cure a variety of conditions when there is as yet no scientific evidence to support the claims. The FDA warns consumers not to abandon conventional medical treatment in favor of products that have no proven value and that claim to be cure-alls.

The cosmetic use of aloe vera falls under a different set of rules. The FDA cannot require that cosmetics manufacturers test their products for safety before they are sold. It can only take action against a product that is adulterated or mislabeled. According to an article in *FDA Consumer,* aloe vera cosmetics have not resulted in any problem.

In addition, the FDA has imposed a policy in recent years that prohibits virtually all support, both financial and otherwise, by drug and medical device manufacturers, to disseminate information about off-label uses of existing FDA-approved drugs or medical devices. The FDA designed the policy to prevent blatant promotion of research findings and results. However, in the summer of 1994, the Washington Legal Foundation, on behalf of research and biotech companies such as Carrington Laboratories in Texas, filed a lawsuit to abolish this policy to further promote the sharing of scientific research and results. The Foundation claims that researchers and medical scientists have been denied their freedom of speech, and at the same time, denied opportunities to share ideas and findings critical in the progress of aloe research. (At the time of this writing, the issue is still not resolved.)

According to medical anthropologist Robert Trotter, aloe vera is a plant, not a controlled substance, so it does not fall under any of the controlled substances acts. "All the FDA can do is determine whether aloe products are labeled correctly.

"Aloe vera could be considered an 'orphan' drug, which means that even though it may be effective, it is not economically feasible for a pharmaceutical company to produce," Dr. Trotter continues. "Orphan drugs have two characteristics: they either treat an illness so rare that pharmaceutical companies don't profit by producing them, or they are derived from natural products which cannot be patented and so are not financially attractive to pharmaceutical companies."

Trotter estimates that it costs between $7 million and $32 million to "proof" a drug to provide the research to back up the claims. Not surprisingly, that type of investment doesn't seem worth while to many companies when others would profit equally from the money they invest in research.

Although patents are issued on the stabilization formulas and other processes used to make aloe vera products, Trotter says that the pure plant extracts cannot be patented. "Once the benefits were proven, anyone could begin selling it without the burden of the start-up costs," Trotter explains. "The new company could produce aloe products and sell them more cheaply, ruining the profitability for the company that did the research."

Some aloe vera businesspeople prefer to see aloe vera gels and juices continue to be classified by the FDA as a health drink and nothing more. They believe that the research being done on aloe vera might hurt the industry if the FDA were to classify aloe vera as a drug, thereby limiting the use of aloe vera products as a natural remedy for a variety of illnesses and diseases.

THE CONTENT CONTROVERSY

In addition to some exaggerated claims, many aloe vera businesspeople say that a few companies stretch the truth about the aloe vera content of their products. "There are a few salespeople who are taking advantage of the situation," remarks Bill Coats. "In the last twenty-three years, I've seen 300 companies come and go because, without quality products, they couldn't repeat sales. You can sell anything one time."

"The consumer must beware of false labeling," cautions Lou Massbauer, distributor of aloe vera products in San Diego, California. "Some products on the market that claim 99 percent aloe vera actually contain less than 10 percent."

Ray Henry concurs: "Many so-called aloe vera products contain only 5 percent pure aloe vera. Since there are no legal regulations, some contain preservatives, bleaching agents, and sweeteners without saying so," he says. "But we can't blame the FDA for not enforcing regulations because, since they can't prove what's in the product, they can't prove false labeling."

Because the stabilization process requires that water and preservatives be added to aloe vera to maintain its efficacy, stabilized aloe vera gels and juices have varying percentages of pure aloe vera in them. Most gels and juices claim to have an aloe vera content just tenths of a percent below 100.

"To determine what real aloe vera gel is like, cut a leaf from a plant, peel it with a cheese cutter, rinse the pulp and liquefy in a blender," suggests McAnalley. "Pour into a glass and observe its appearance and taste. That's what 100 percent aloe vera gel looks like—even though the nature of the gel varies from harvest to harvest."

Smothers says consumers will know if a product has a high

aloe vera content because they'll be able to taste it and smell it. If a product doesn't have much taste at all, it's probably diluted. "Don't just look at the front of the label where the word 'aloe' is plastered all over," cautions Smothers. "Look at the ingredient label where ingredients are listed by concentration. If aloe vera is the last ingredient on the label, there's only a small amount present. If it's within the first two to four items, the product probably has significant amounts of aloe vera."

Smothers suggests that consumers also look for the use of aloe vera extract, which usually denotes a diluted product. "I've seen products that list aloe vera extracts as the first ingredient. That means that they may say they have 45 or 50 percent of this extract in there but the extract may only be 5 percent aloe vera to start with."

Another term to note is "reconstituted aloe vera," which, according to Smothers, means that the aloe vera has been reconstituted from a powder or concentrated as a liquid. "In my opinion, either process decreases the efficacy of the product," he says. "Some people think that reconstituted aloe vera is fine, but consumers should be aware that they are buying that type of product."

According to Smothers, the NASC created a list of definitions for the various aspects of aloe vera because so many different terms are used throughout the industry (see Appendix A). "By using standard terms, we will all be reading off the same sheet of music," Smothers says. "It's taken some time for people in the aloe vera industry to break old habits, but by using the same terms we are beginning to understand each other better."

McAnalley cautions consumers about aloe vera products that advertise "No preservatives added." "Aloe has to be preserved or it will decompose," he explains. "We've tested some products that claim to have no preservatives and they did have them. One reason this may occur is that the company who bottles the product doesn't put preservatives in it but the company which supplied them the aloe vera did."

CAN STANDARDS FOR ALOE VERA BE SET?

To date, the aloe vera industry has not agreed upon a set of standards by which products can be evaluated. Therefore, the claims made for the aloe vera content in products and the testing performed vary from company to company.

It might seem that the percentage of aloe vera in a product could be based simply on the ratio of pure aloe vera from the leaf to additives, but not all aloe vera plants have the same biochemistry. The moisture content of a plant that has been growing in an area drenched by rain for days before the harvest will be much higher than that of a plant that has been growing in a drought area. Similarly, a plant that has been sitting on a loading dock for days before being shipped and processed will probably have a different water content than one that is processed immediately after harvesting.

Because of these differences in moisture content, many believe that the percentage of aloe is best judged by measuring the content of solids found in the plant. "Other products—including orange juice and milk—present the same type of dilemma," says Smothers. "The phosphates, lactates, lactylates, and butterfat in milk may vary depending on the food and water fed to the cattle. The milk industry came up with a standard of measuring butterfat and decided that to be called whole milk, a product must contain a certain percentage of butterfat."

"You would think that any cow would produce 100 percent milk, but when you sell a food, government agencies have to have some standards by which to measure quality," adds Howard. "Aloe vera businesses do not define 100 percent aloe vera based on what comes out of the leaf, necessarily, but on solid ingredients in the leaf, such as the calcium and magnesium. When manufacturers buy leaves from the farmers, peel them and put [them] into products, they need to measure the quality of the aloe vera so that they know how much of it to use. But I would venture to guess that, because of the cost of testing, 95 percent of the aloe vera sold in this country is tested solely for bacterial contamination and not for content," says Howard.

In an effort to standardize the testing for aloe vera content throughout the industry, Carrington Laboratories spent over $100,000 to develop a method for quality control testing, according to Howard. "We analyzed over fifty chemical ingredients in aloe vera gel from leaves harvested each month for more than a year to establish a chemical profile of an 'average' leaf," says Howard. "We used this method to analyze commercial products being sold during mid-1982, and were shocked to find that a number of commercial products labeled 100 percent aloe vera were found to be 5, 10, 15, 20, and 30 percent aloe vera. We printed the results in a consumer report to alert the public and the aloe industry to the need for correction because we knew that if the industry didn't put a stop to mislabeling, the government would."

Howard says that because it would be too costly for companies to test for fifty ingredients on each aloe vera sample for routine quality control, Carrington Laboratories developed a method to test for only four ingredients as a routine procedure. "The simplified method we developed would work on fresh and preserved aloe vera gel for in-house testing in factory laboratories where the preservatives used in the product were known," explains Howard. "But the test was not adequate for investigative purposes by an outside laboratory in which the preservatives were not known because the types of preservative used could affect the aloe vera content reading."

"At first it looked like our method would be adopted by the NASC," continues Howard. "The Science and Technical Committee of the NASC submitted our method to outside laboratories and it received excellent confirmation. The NASC also announced adoption of the Avacare method in an official news release, and the findings were published in trade journals. But certain NASC members did not like the fact that Avacare got the publicity for funding the study. The NASC denied that the method for testing aloe vera adopted by the NASC was the same that we had developed. When we saw the letter, we protested, [but] they weren't willing to do anything about it, so we left the NASC."

Smothers says that the Carrington Laboratories analysis looked promising to the NASC, but they did not adopt it because they felt that the analytical procedures could not be easily reproduced by others. "Carrington Laboratories' method of assaying the product did not always work in labs with inadequate equipment, but labs with good equipment have reproduced the test," he explains.

Smothers adds that when the NASC tested aloe vera for fifty ingredients, the results fluctuated dramatically, but the NASC has determined that there are four constituents that seem to fluctuate in harmony with each other. They include total solids, calcium, magnesium, and the HPLC (high pressure liquid chromatography) ratio. "When one is high, the others will all be high; when one is low, all the others will be low," says Smothers. "And if one reading is extremely high relative to the others, we can determine if someone is trying to spike the results."

Although some preservatives can cause a discrepancy in the HPLC reading, testing for all four constituents provides a more reliable aloe vera content assessment than simply testing for the HPLC ratio. Common preservatives approved for aloe vera food products are sodium benzoate and potassium sorbate. Methyl paraben is used as a preservative for topically applied aloe vera. Citric acid and ascorbic acid act as buffering agents to help maintain the pH balance of aloe vera products.

"Based on this research, the NASC Science and Technical Committee has come up with a new analytical profile to define what can be called 100 percent aloe vera," says Smothers. "Our goal is to have all aloe vera companies include information on their product labels and promotional material about how their product compares to NASC standards."

Smothers says the NASC is using that formula to institute a system whereby a company that markets a product containing aloe vera can apply to the NASC to have their product certified. "We will employ an outside laboratory to investigate that product and then certify that the product does or does not meet the claims on the label," he explains. "That way we can make our opinion known and that will go a long way toward enabling people to have more confidence in the aloe vera content of a product. The product would have a seal of approval like the Underwriter's Laboratory or *Good Housekeeping* seal.

"We have two of the largest aloe vera product companies in the country who want to have their products certified. By doing so it will put pressure on other people in the business. If that happens, people who are making unsupported claims will clean up their act. Other companies might ignore it but their products might eventually be ignored by the public. Then they'd either quit using the words 'aloe vera' to market their products or put enough in there to make their claims correct," says Smothers.

As a trade association the NASC is not a policing agency, and use of the analytical procedure to evaluate products will be left up to individual companies in the membership. Additionally, Smothers says that the NASC hopes to create a certification process for testing products.

"The primary goal of the NASC is to conduct joint scientific research, attempt to unravel some of the mysteries of aloe vera, and make order out of chaos within the industry," says Smothers. "Though we know much more than when we started, there's still a lot we don't know.

"Organizing the NASC has been difficult," Smothers continues. "Many members of the association are also competitors, each with their own interests to protect, but even though their companies may be extremely competitive, many of our members have learned to work together. It has been serendipitous that people who were formerly so antagonistic and who had reservations about one another have become working associates within our organization."

However, the NASC has had its share of controversy, and membership has dwindled over the past few years. Some companies have dropped out from the NASC because they couldn't live up to the code of ethics; others left because they disagreed with the premise of regulating the industry. Membership has also dwindled as companies are forced out of business. Some in the aloe vera industry believe that FDA regulations, the NASC standards, competition, and two freezes in the Rio Grande Valley in recent years have all had an impact on the selling of aloe vera and may serve, in the long term, to reduce the number of people who remain in the business.

"I am optimistic about aloe vera's future, but believe that firms that sell inferior products or exaggerate their effectiveness will not stay in business," says Jerome N. Michell, chairman of the board of Fruit of the Earth, an aloe vera product distribution company in Bensenville, Illinois. "I think eventually the aloe vera business will settle down to a half a dozen to a dozen legitimate companies, and I think they will enjoy a good-selling product for a long time."

A Balm
for Burns

Fred and Judy Cook of La Mesa, California, and their seven-year-old daughter, Suzanne, were enjoying dinner at a local Chinese restaurant one evening when suddenly Suzanne dropped a cup of hot tea into her lap, severely burning her leg. Judy immediately called the family pediatrician, who suggested applying a pharmaceutical ointment to the burn and wrapping the leg in gauze.

"The wound was a mess the next morning," Judy recalls. "Suzanne had been wearing a polyester skirt, and the hot tea melted the material onto her leg. When we lifted the bandage her skin came off. It was a raw, weepy wound, and I was upset with the doctor for recommending that treatment."

That day, a customer who frequented one of the health food stores owned by the Cooks gave the family some leaves from her aloe vera plant to help heal the burn. Where the prescribed ointment failed, aloe vera gel succeeded.

"For three or four days we treated the burn with gel straight from the plant," says Judy. "Today Suzanne doesn't even have a scar on her leg."

According to Judy, aloe vera's healing power was what convinced her and Fred to become distributors and, ultimately, general managers of Forever Living Products, a line of aloe vera health and beauty items.

Like the Cooks, thousands of people nationwide, including many medical practitioners, are convinced that the aloe vera gel and juice contain restorative properties that can be beneficial for all types of thermal burns (injuries caused by temperature changes), including radiation burns, sunburn, and frostbite. They believe that the plant contains an enzymatic property that helps the burn to heal, keeps wounds clean, and lowers the risk of infection.

STUDIES SHOW HOW ALOE HEALS BURNS

Although the FDA has not concurred on the plant's attributes for anything but minor first-aid measures, several university studies have documented aloe vera's medicinal powers in treating severe burns and frostbite.

Research conducted at the University of Chicago Hospital and Wayne State University in Detroit, by John P. Heggers, Ph.D., Martin C. Robson, M.D., and other researchers, has shown that using an aloe-based cream to treat thermal injuries can retard the effects of the burn and revitalize damaged skin cells.

According to Dr. Heggers, director of research for the Division of Plastic and Reconstructive Surgery at Wayne State University, burn injuries are not uniform in their damage. "If you look at a burn wound, the tissue in the center receives the most heat, which coagulates protein and kills skin tissue," he explains. "The adjacent tissue is partially injured, and if not treated will die within twenty-four to forty-eight hours."

Dr. Heggers goes on to explain that when skin tissue is injured certain components called prostaglandins and thromboxanes are liberated. The thromboxane is what researchers believe to be the prime mediator of progressive cell death after a thermal injury.

We searched for a product that would prevent the partially damaged tissue from dying and found success with a cream called Dermaide Aloe," says Dr. Heggers. "This product is a mixture of 70 percent aloe vera extract combined with a pharmaceutical cream base.

"We treated 154 cases of frostbite. Fifty-six were treated with aloe vera and only seven percent had some type of infection. Of the 98 patients who were not treated with aloe vera, 33 percent needed amputation.

"We believe that the active ingredient in aloe vera probably acts as a substrate inhibitor, which means it binds the enzyme system together to prevent the production of thromboxane. We are now conducting clinical studies of the cream's effect on burn patients."

According to Dr. Heggers, the first studies he and his colleagues conducted were corroborated by Neil S. Pennies, M.D., from the University of Miami Medical School: "Dr. Pennies' research affirmed that aloe vera extract has a tremendous inhibitory effect in preventing the production of the mediators of progressive dermal necrosis."

While Dr. Heggers has seen that aloe vera helps heal burns, he stresses that a special concentration of the aloe juice extract, not the gel, is needed to be effective. "I have not experimented with using the fresh plant on burns, so I cannot say whether or not it is effective," he stresses. "I am talking as a scientist, not as a faith healer. I have looked at some aloe vera products on the market today, but they are not made in the concentration that we recommend for treating thermal injuries. Our aloe is a dermaide aloe processed by Aloe-Shere of Dallas and mixed with a pharmaceutical cream base, which has standard component factors in it that compare with any of the other topical creams that are used in treating thermal injury."

REDUCING SCARRING

Aloe speeds up the healing process of burns, stimulates the growth of healthy skin cells, and limits the body's production of scar tissue. According to Elizabeth Burdick, M.S., a microbiologist and skin therapist who treats burn trauma patients at Dermatherapy, Inc., in Encinitas, California, scar tissue is thick like a callus and is produced by basal cells that are found in the last layer of the derma. "When the skin is burned or traumatized in some other way, the body sends a message to the basal cells to help protect it," explains Burdick. "Within twenty-four hours, the basal cells travel up to the epidermal layer and produce a scab. Underneath the scab, keratinized tissue forms, which is thick scar tissue created to protect the body from trauma."

According to Burdick, aloe interferes with the process of scar formation. "We don't know exactly what the mechanism is, but somehow the aloe vera causes skin cells to regenerate so rapidly that the body does not send the message to the basal cells. The new epidermal skin cells begin closing off the injured area. While the body will still produce a scab-like covering, it doesn't have a thick, rough texture to it. Underneath the scab is healthy skin tissue, not keratinized tissue or scar tissue."

Taking the Sting Out of Sunburn

The main cause of sunburn is UV-B radiation (ultraviolet B rays), which can cause pain in the short term and promote aging and sometimes even skin cancer in the long term. The body's natural weapon against ultraviolet radiation is the skin pigment melanin. Acting as a defensive barricade, melanin absorbs and disperses ultraviolet radiation away from the skin.

If a person's true skin color is already dark, there is more melanin on the top layers of skin. The more melanin the better, but it still does not insure the skin against the sun's harmful rays.

Many sunscreens on the market contain chemicals that disperse the UV-B rays in a similar way to melanin. Several of them also include aloe vera to help moisturize dry, damaged skin.

Steve Finley, former president of Burn-Off Corporation in Irving, Texas, says that people burn for two reasons—the effect of the ultraviolet rays and dehydration of the skin. "To protect against burning," says Finley, "we include three sunscreens in our sunblock product. To keep the skin moisturized, we add 61 percent pure aloe gel."

While Finley believes that aloe isn't a necessary ingredient in sun blocks, he says it's essential to include in burn relief products. "Too many ultraviolet rays and too much wind and sun exposure cause the skin to dehydrate," he says. "Most products don't attack both problems.

Finley says that when he first produced his product six years ago, he tested the formula on 100 people in Cozumel, Mexico. "Many Texans and mid-westerners go to Cozumel to scuba dive," explains Finley, "and most everyone gets sunburned. I gave samples of Burn-Off to 100 people, and every one who tried it said it eliminated the pain and restored moisture to their dehydrated skin."

One woman from Atlanta, Georgia, who used Burn-Off products to treat sunburn, wrote to Finley: "For the first time in my life, I experienced neither itching nor peeling after long exposure to the sun."

Another woman from Mineral Wells, Texas, said that her husband burned the tops of his feet so badly that they blistered and swelled. After he used The Green Stuff, one of Burn-Off's aloe vera products, the pain and swelling subsided, "and he could wear shoes the very next day," she wrote.

A HOME REMEDY FOR BURNS

For thousands of years, people have relied on aloe vera to doctor burns—from mild sunburns to more serious burns. By applying the gel to the wound, they have not only been relieved of pain but have also prevented scarring and blisters.

Today, the aloe vera plant is still used as a first aid treatment for burns. Even though many people have seen wonderful results from using fresh gel from the plant, some physicians and aloe vera manufacturers warn against that use and say there are safer ways to derive the plant's benefits.

"Any skin product that incorporates aloe should be processed," says Burdick. "Aloe gel taken directly from the plant is not sterile and may contain bacteria which can create complications when working with an open wound like a burn. I'd recommend using a sterile aloe vera–based burn salve."

If you choose to use the gel straight from the leaf, you'll get the best results from a plant over three years of age. Snip off a large leaf, cutting as near to the stem as you can. Wash the cutting thoroughly and remove the sharp spines of the leaf's sides with a sharp knife. Then slice the leaf down the middle.

Some people apply the sliced-open aloe leaf directly on the burn. Others allow the aloe vera gel to drain from the leaf into a container to try to keep the gel as free as possible of the yellow sap, which can irritate a burn. They then soak a bandage in the gel and wrap the bandage around the burn. Still others combine these two techniques by placing the cut piece of leaf on the wound and covering it with a bandage; the bandage then remains moist and does not cling to the wound.

TREATING THE SKIN WITH ALOE VERA 7

As the largest organ in the human body, the skin accounts for 16 percent of the body's total weight. In a male of average size, the surface area of his skin measures over 2,800 square inches. Tough as it may seem, human skin is sensitive to the effects of heat and cold and is often subjected to injury, infection, and irritation. Aloe vera juice and gel have proved helpful in treating many types of skin problems, including insect bites, rashes, stings, dry-chapped skin, abrasions, fever blisters, diaper rash, razor burns, and fungal infections.

According to Bill Coats, R.Ph., of Coats Aloe International, aloe vera used topically kills bacteria and viruses, such as the herpes simplex virus, which causes fever blisters and cold sores, and the herpes zoster virus, which causes shingles. It also stimulates healing. Studies performed by Bill Wolfe, D.D.S., also show that aloe vera inhibits the growth of these viruses.

One woman in Ontario, Canada, has seen first-hand how aloe vera cures cold sores. A testimonial letter she wrote to the

Burn-Off Corporation explains that she used a Burn-Off sun-burn relief product as soon as she felt a cold sore developing. "Right away, it numbed the cold sore so it did not hurt," she says. "In a few days, the sore disappeared without ever break-ing into an actual cold sore."

A woman from Carson City, Nevada, can attest to aloe vera's role in healing shingles. In a letter to American Dream International, Inc., a multi-level aloe vera marketing company in Visalia, California, she said that her uncle developed shingles after having his leg amputated. Antibiotics and other prescribed drugs had failed to cure the condition, so the woman began bathing the affected areas with American Dream International's aloe-based Bath and Shower Gelee, applying jojoba oil and then applying aloe vera gel. In addition, her uncle drank three ounces of aloe vera juice before each meal. By the second day, the shingles began to improve. By the seventh day, all but a couple of sores had disappeared, and within a month he was completely healed.

"As an anti-inflammatory agent, aloe vera dissolves dead, devitalized cells like those found in decubitus ulcers and bed-sores," says Coats. "Initially, aloe vera may cause the sore to deepen and enlarge because it is working its way past the dead tissue to help heal the live tissue."

Coats relates the story of Danny Choo, a man in Malaysia who sought relief for severe ulcerations of his lower leg caused by an accident ten years earlier. "The Kiwanians wanted to send Choo to the United States so I could treat him with aloe vera," says Coats. "I told them the trip wasn't necessary, and instead sent aloe vera products and instructions on how to use them to treat the ulcers. I suggested that Choo put his foot in a pan and use a wash cloth to rinse aloe vera juice over his ulcerated leg for thirty minutes twice a day. I also recommended that he rub the ulcer wounds with aloe vera jelly every three hours."

The aloe vera treatment proved so effective that within sixty days all the dead debris in the wound was gone. "I recently received a thank-you letter from Choo, saying that his leg was almost completely healed," says Coats. "Sometimes aloe vera works when other things don't."

Anne Ayers of Montgomery, Alabama, agrees. She became interested in aloe vera products when they healed her mother's painful and persistent bedsores. "My mother began using a bottle of aloe vera lotion and within a week the bedsores were gone," says Ayers.

Others have also found aloe vera effective for healing bedsores. A nursing home in Texas began using a sunburn relief and moisturizing product called The Green Stuff made by Burn-Off Corporation on decubitus ulcers and bedsores. "Our product is 98 percent aloe vera gel plus thickeners and preservatives," says Steve Finley, Burn-Off's founder and former president. "We didn't know it would work on bedsores, but the nurses told us that it does a better job on early stage bedsores than any other product. Today many nursing homes in Texas are using the product."

Some people have claimed that aloe vera juice can cure skin cancer when used regularly over several months. Art Benson, a Carrington Laboratories distributor from North Hollywood, California tells his story: "My brother, a longshoreman in Seattle, Washington, had been through several operations for skin cancer of the face. Finally, he used aloe vera cream and it cured him. He started selling aloe vera products to the other longshoremen and eventually the longshoremen's union suggested aloe vera's use to its members. Today, there's almost no skin cancer on the Seattle waterfront."

But aloe vera doesn't work on all skin cancer. While some people have experienced personal success using aloe to treat sunburn and arthritis pain, others have experienced no benefit in using it to treat skin cancers.

That wouldn't surprise Norman Orentreich, M.D., professor of dermatology at the New York University Medical School and a practicing dermatologist for over thirty-five years. "A lot of people claim that aloe vera cures everything—hair loss, ingrown toenails, burns, and arthritis. Our experience has shown that aloe vera makes a soothing, wet compress, but there are many substances that are soothing when applied to inflamed, irritated skin. Water with the right ingredients in it—like milk or oils—is soothing. But a wet compress does not help warts, acne, or psoriasis."

In contrast, Max B. Skousen, Director of the Aloe Vera Research Institute in West Valley City, Utah, and author of *The Ancient Egyptian Medicine Plant: Aloe Vera Handbook*, finds that aloe vera helps fight skin breakouts. He offers a three-step process in using aloe vera to treat acne. First, cleanse the face morning and night. Then apply aloe vera juice or gel and let it dry. This acts as an astringent to reduce oily skin and also stimulates the tissue to heal without scarring. Finally, he suggests using aloe vera ointment directly on pimples and other sores to enhance healing and reduce the possibility of scarring.

James Fulton, M.D., a dermatologist from Newport Beach, California, uses aloe vera to treat his patients. "Any wound we treat, whether it's suturing a cut or removing a skin cancer, heals better with aloe vera on it," he says.

Dr. Fulton centrifuges aloe vera juice to remove particles, combines the juice with Aloe Activator (a Forever Living product), soaks the surgical dressing in the solution, and applies it to the wound. He instructs patients to change the dressing every twelve hours. "Using this solution cuts the healing time in half," he says.

Although Dr. Fulton does not currently use aloe vera to treat acne, he is developing an aloe vera ice to help reduce acne inflammation and hasten healing. "The acne sufferer will first cleanse the area with benzol peroxide scrub cleanser, then use the ice as a compress for five minutes, and wash the area again," explains Dr. Fulton. "This is not a treatment in itself, but an adjunct which increases the effectiveness of the regular treatment."

It is difficult to say what percentage of the dermatologists endorses the use of aloe vera to combat acne. The approach that many dermatologists seem to take is "If my patients find that it works, great, but I don't use it in my practice."

Though physicians may prefer other forms of treatment, many people are more comfortable using natural products and have seen positive results from using aloe vera to help heal all types of skin irritations, from cuts and scrapes to skin ulcers and burns.

THE BEAUTY OF ALOE: ALOE VERA IN SKIN AND HAIR PRODUCTS 8

A miraculous innovation for reducing wrinkles. A cure-all for spotty, blotchy skin; dry patches; and sunburn. A natural cleanser and conditioner for hair. Such superlatives cannot be used without arousing the ire of the FDA, but many skin and hair care experts agree that aloe vera contains certain emollients and healing properties that improve the skin, scalp, and hair.

Aloe vera's value as a skin softener dates back to ancient history, and even today many aestheticians and skin therapists regard it as an important ingredient of skin care products.

"A lot of things that are considered a fad today were used thousands of years ago by the Egyptians and North and Central American Indians," says Rachel Perry, owner of Rachel Perry Cosmetics in Chatsworth, California, and author of *Reverse the Aging Process of Your Face*. "For years no one used aloe vera, but in the 1970s it was rediscovered. Aloe is good for the skin because it restores the skin to its natural pH balance and gives skin a smoother appearance."

"Aloe vera and clay are two of my favorite ingredients because they are both from the earth and both can be taken internally," Perry continues. "Aloe vera juice is good for cleansing, and a glass of it diluted with water draws toxins out of the body."

Whether aloe vera helps the skin and hair in the myriad of ways purported is yet to be proved. Thus far, respected scientific journals have documented claims relating only to the emollient, moisturizing, and healing properties of the gel—the part of the plant used to make skin and hair care products.

The properties found in aloe gel are attributed to complex carbohydrates known as polysaccharides. Many believe that when the polysaccharides combine with other substances present in the gel, they create a synergistic effect that accounts for aloe vera's beneficial effects.

Used alone, the astringent properties in aloe vera tend to dry out the skin, but because aloe has the ability to penetrate the skin, many say it is an excellent ingredient to incorporate into moisturizers. As Elizabeth Burdick, a biochemist, skin therapist, and co-owner of Dermatherapy, Inc., in Encinitas, California, says, "Aloe vera has wonderful healing effects but it can be excessively drying. Products containing aloe vera need to include humectants that will buffer aloe's drying effects."

According to Bill Coats, R.Ph., author of *The Silent Healer,* the surface oils found in most cosmetics are effective only when they are on the skin. When they evaporate or are wiped off, the benefit ends. But aloe vera permeates all three layers of the skin.

"One reason aloe vera penetrates the skin is because it actually lowers the surface tension of water," explains Don Smothers. "For example, if you place a steel needle on top of a glass filled with water, the needle will float because of the surface tension of the water. If you put something in the water that lowers the tension, the needle will sink. Aloe is a substance that lowers surface tension of water, even though it's primarily comprised of water."

When used as a cosmetic ingredient, aloe's penetrating abilities permit water and other moisturizing agents to submerge into the skin to replenish fluids. As it penetrates, the hyaluronic acids present in aloe sink deeply into the skin, removing toxins and allowing the astringent properties of the plant to work in a more effective manner.

"A lot of moisture lotions keep the skin from losing moisture. Aloe does that plus it pulls moisture out of the air and takes it into the skin," comments Bill McAnalley, former vice president and research director of Carrington Laboratories, who is also a licensed cosmetologist.

Aloe vera helps to keep facial pores unclogged and gives skin a healthy glow because the enzymatic activity in the plant speeds up the blood circulation and sloughs off dead skin. The amino acids in the plant then help to promote the growth of new cells. Additionally, aloe vera furnishes the skin with a protective coating to help retard the growth of harmful bacteria and fungi.

The astringent properties of the plant's gel counteract acne infection and help cure blemishes with little or no scarring. Because aloe vera has an acidic pH factor similar to that of the skin, it helps to restore the skin to its natural pH. "The pH of the skin varies from pH4 to pH6," explains Ray Henry, a former senior vice president of Aloe Laboratories of Texas. "Aloe's natural pH is about 4.3, depending on weather and soil conditions, so it's very close to that of human skin."

As with any skin treatment, aloe vera users must be patient. Some people plagued with acne report that before their skin condition improves, they get worse because impurities are made to surface. But when they follow a regular routine using aloe vera products, their skin improves.

"I've used aloe vera for three years, not only for bites and burns but for skin eruptions," says Geri Wilson from Burlington, Massachusetts. "When my face breaks out, I wash it and put aloe vera cream on before I go to bed. Within a week's time my skin will have cleared up. Aloe vera is not magic, but it helps to promote healing."

"The most essential part of any skin care program is keeping the skin clean," says Elizabeth Burdick. "Remember, the skin is an excretory organ and residue must be removed for healthy skin. I recommend that women, men, and children wash their face every morning when they wake up and every evening before they go to bed and that they wash twice each time; the first cleansing removes surface debris, the second removes other impurities in the skin."

After the face is clean, Burdick suggests applying a balancing solution in the form of a toner. "This can be a commercial product or diluted witch hazel," she says. "After toning, the skin should be moisturized not only to make the skin more subtle but to protect it from the sun, wind, and air pollutants."

After the moisturizer has penetrated the skin, Burdick recommends applying a sunblock with a sun protection factor (SPF) of twelve or higher. "I suggest using a sunblock every day because even when it's cloudy, the sun's ultraviolet rays can damage the skin."

She also recommends applying a facial masque every

month to remove the dead cells and promote new cell growth.

Whether you're working to improve your hair or your skin, skin therapists and hairdressers alike will insist that a creamy complexion and a lustrous head of hair start from the inside out. A healthy diet and a regular exercise program are essential ingredients of any beauty plan.

"A balanced diet of fruits, vegetables, proteins, and carbohydrates is essential for healthy skin," Burdick says. "In addition, I suggest drinking four to eight glasses of purified water each day—not tap water or mineral water. The skin is a waste removal organ that protects our body and controls our body temperature. Water helps to remove toxins from the body, and if we don't get enough, the skin looks blotchy, dark circles form under the eyes, and breakouts are more apt to occur."

PROMOTING HEALTHIER HAIR

In addition to improving the skin, aloe vera works equally well on the hair and scalp. When incorporated into shampoos with other appropriate ingredients, aloe's deep-penetrating ability opens the scalp's pores. As it penetrates the scalp, the plant's amino acids help to revitalize healthy tissue. The aloe vera then helps to thoroughly cleanse the scalp and brings impurities to the surface, so they can be rinsed away.

Aloe vera also serves as a good hair conditioning agent because it penetrates the hair shaft. Keratin, the primary protein of hair, consists of amino acids, oxygen, carbon, and small amounts of hydrogen, nitrogen, and sulfur. Aloe vera has a chemical make-up similar to that of keratin, and it rejuvenates the hair with its own nutrients, giving it more elasticity and preventing breakage.

Vernon Pruitt, president of the Terry Corporation, a private label aloe vera product company in Melbourne, Florida, says research indicates that aloe vera is beneficial in shampoos, rinses, and conditioners because it is substantive to the hair, meaning that it remains in contact with the hair shaft.

Pruitt maintains that because aloe vera is beneficial to the skin it also helps the scalp. But since most people leave shampoo on their hair for a short time and the shower water dilutes the shampoo, Pruitt recommends using a heavier concentration of aloe vera shampoo to treat the scalp. "Or try a two-part system," he suggests: "Use a lesser concentration of aloe vera shampoo and leave an aloe conditioner on the hair for three to five minutes."

Like new skin care regimens, new hair care programs take time to prove their effectiveness. People trying aloe vera hair products are cautioned against expecting overnight results.

SELECTING ALOE BEAUTY PRODUCTS

Aloe vera's name recognition and appeal among consumers of beauty products was demonstrated in 1981 when *Glamour* and *Self* magazines each conducted telephone surveys of 200 people. According to Vernon Pruitt of the Terry Corporation, the survey participants were asked to rate how the following ingredients influenced their buying habits: aloe vera, jojoba, vitamins E and F, collagen, conditioners, natural soluble protein, cell-renewal ingredients, sunscreen, natural ingredients, and hypo-allergenics.

"Aloe vera placed number three in order of importance, just after vitamins E and F and 'natural ingredients'," says Pruitt. "In the second survey people were asked simply if they were aware of the following scientific ingredients in skin care products: aloe vera, vitamins, elastin, collagen, sodium RNA, linoleic acid, mucopolysaccharide, and jojoba. In this survey, aloe vera came out second to vitamins. Of those surveyed 80 percent were aware that vitamins were used as an ingredient in skin care products and 77.5 percent were aware of aloe vera."

It's because of high name recognition and consumer demand that some cosmetics firms have added only token amounts of aloe vera to their products in order to say that they have the benefits. Ingredients are listed in descending order of their quantity, so be sure to check the list of ingredients on the label. If the aloe vera in drinks and gels is not at or near the top of the list, it is probably in such small amounts as to be of little value.

Don't think, though, that aloe vera–containing cosmetics are effective only if they contain high percentages of the plant extract. Unlike aloe vera drinks, most say more is not better where cosmetics are concerned.

Most people agree that a high percentage of pure aloe vera is most effective when taken internally or used externally to heal disease or injury, whereas many aloe vera cosmetics manufacturers say that too high a concentration of the plant in cosmetics can dry out the skin.

"When we started in business fifteen years ago, people asked 'What's aloe vera?' Now they ask, 'How much aloe vera is in the product?'" says Frank Romano, president of Key West Aloe in Florida, which sells bath, hair, suntan, cosmetic, and men's grooming products made with aloe vera. "It has become a numbers game, and that's a problem. The efficacy of certain products—especially cosmetics—does not depend on the percentage of aloe vera but on 'aloe genetics,' a term we've coined to say it takes the right ingredients combined with the right amount of aloe vera to do the job."

As an ingredient in moisturizers, aloe vera gel should account for at least 3 percent by weight of the product to benefit the skin, according to General Nutrition Mills, Inc., a subsidiary of General Nutrition Incorporated, which manufacturers aloe vera products at its Fargo, North Dakota, facility.

McAnalley says Carrington Laboratories has seen good results in skin care with products that contain as little as 15 to 20 percent aloe vera. "Skin care products seem to work with anywhere from 15 to 99 percent, depending on whether you have oily or dry skin," he says.

Elizabeth Burdick says that she does not use more than 18 percent aloe vera in her products. "In my products, aloe vera is used as a vehicle to carry nutrients into the skin," she explains. "If I include too much aloe vera, it tends to counteract the other enzymes I use in my products."

Some purists use aloe vera directly from the leaf as a healing masque for skin problems. A popular woman's magazine suggests tossing a leaf into a blender to liquefy it, then applying the liquid to the skin for ten minutes before rinsing it off with water. While this homemade remedy might be effective to dry up skin breakouts, applying fresh aloe vera as a cosmetic is not generally recommended by skin specialists or product manufacturers.

McAnalley warns that it's difficult for most people at home to remove the gel from the plant without contaminating it with the plant's yellow sap. "In our research, we've found that aloe vera stimulates the growth of human cells, but that the latex or yellow sap kills cells. This is why people should be careful about using house plants for cosmetic purposes or to treat burns."

ALOE SELLS COSMETICS

In recent years, many cosmetics firms have climbed on the aloe vera bandwagon, offering a wide array of sunscreens, moisturizers, night creams, and shampoos to meet perceived or actual consumer demand.

A spokesman for Chesebrough Ponds, which distributes Vaseline Brand Intensive Care Lotion, admits that his firm added the Herbal & Aloe lotion to its product line "because of strong demand and competition from the other companies in the marketplace."

After the green-bottled liquid made its debut in July 1983, sales of Vaseline Brand Intensive Care Lotion increased for the first twelve to fifteen months, he said. Thereafter, they stabilized to their current market share, which he declined to identify. However, sales of the Herbal & Aloe Intensive Care Lotion remain below those of the original lotion, which has been sold for years.

Dr. Paul Koehler, a former medical director at Chesebrough Ponds, Inc., emphasizes that his company makes no claim for miraculous, curative powers in its aloe vera product. "There's not anything exceedingly scientific or novel in our incorporating aloe vera in our Herbal and Aloe Vaseline Brand Intensive Care Lotion," he says. "It was done to make the product more contemporary and give it a little pizzazz."

Koehler adds that aloe vera has been known for years to act as a moisturizer and emollient and to have wound or skin healing effects, "but these claims have not been substantiated by well-controlled studies."

Health food stores throughout the country abound with numerous brands of aloe-containing cosmetics. Greentree

Grocers, a health food store in San Diego, California, offers gels, shampoos, creams, moisturizers, sunscreens, and other cosmetics manufactured by companies like Lily of the Desert, Natureade, Nature's Gate, Rich Life, Mill Creek, and Country Road.

Cosmetics manager and buyer Evan Healy says that all brands are selling well. "I haven't noticed any breakthroughs in the last year or so. The market has pretty much stabilized," says Healy, who uses aloe vera products herself to soften her skin and heal sunburn.

Jerome N. Michell, chairman of the board for Fruit of the Earth in Bensenville, Illinois, says that his company markets its aloe vera products worldwide and that the best-selling cosmetic products are the gel, dry skin cream, and dry skin lotion.

General Nutrition Mills, Inc., in Fargo, North Dakota, indicates that its aloe vera cosmetics are selling well throughout the country. The company recently started an international operation to sell aloe vera products, including cosmetics. According to a company spokesman, three of the company's best sellers are an aloe vera gel, a moisturizing cream, and an aloe/vitamin E skin oil. He emphasizes that although General Nutrition is proud of its aloe vera product line, the company cannot and does not make any claims for medically related benefits. "But by putting aloe vera into products, the consumer gets the benefit of aloe in the cosmetic," he says. "I think it's much more beneficial to a consumer than other vegetable or plant derivatives, even though we don't know what specific ingredient in aloe vera makes it so effective."

Without the scientific studies to back the products, those who sell aloe vera cosmetics through stores or multi-level marketing distribution must depend on testimonials to sell skin and hair care products.

"A good grade aloe vera is worth its weight in gold," says Mary Wilson of Carson City, Nevada, who sells American Dream International, Inc., aloe vera products. "I've been using Ja Lara skin products on my face and they really have helped me from aging. I'm fifty-two years old, and I sell products just on my appearance."

Even people who do not sell aloe vera skin and hair products speak favorably of them. "In all the time I've used aloe vera products on my patrons, not one has ever had an adverse reaction, and many of them have had quite a few benefits," says Lance Ghiorso, a cosmetologist and make-up artist in the La Costa, California, area. The benefits, he added, include glowing, smoother, softer skin, and shiny hair.

Practicing what he preaches, Ghiorso uses a shampoo and weekly facial masque that contain aloe vera ingredients. He also drinks a daily ration of the plant's juice: "It helps my digestive system and gives me more energy."

Ghiorso generally uses commercially prepared substances containing aloe vera, but Julie Russell, a skin care hygienist at the Purple Plum in Encinitas, California, often takes the gel directly from the plant to treat sunburn and other skin irritations. Specializing in body hair removal for women, Russell applies the gel on a client's face, legs, or bikini line after treatment to prevent skin irritation and inflammation.

Like Ghiorso, she also uses creams, moisturizers, and masques that contain aloe vera for facials and other skin care treatments, including foot care. "Aloe is very soothing to the toes and helps to moisten dry, rough feet," she says. "Even though I know that aloe vera's effectiveness has not been proven medically, I believe it really does have healing properties."

Dermatologist Norman Orentreich, M.D., a professor at the New York University Medical School, contends that aloe vera's only benefit is that it is a soothing, moist material. "Aloe vera is no more effective than other gels," he states, "and there is nothing in aloe vera that makes it unique in its ability to soothe or retain water.

Still, people who use aloe products regularly like them. After using The Green Stuff, a 98 percent aloe vera product, for sunburn relief, a woman from Atlanta, Georgia, wrote: "Then I tried The Green Stuff on the laugh lines and wrinkles on my face in an effort to restore the moisture that no other lotion or cream has succeeded in doing. I couldn't believe the difference. Now, after four weeks of using it twice a day, there's been a 90 percent improvement in the lines on my forty-year-old face."

Suzanne Jackson, of San Diego, California, is an avid fan of the plant. "Aloe vera penetrates the skin really well and it's never greasy," she says. "It's not a good moisturizer by itself; it must be mixed with other emollients. But because it penetrates so fast it carries the vitamin E or other moisturizer directly into the skin. People are always guessing that I'm ten years younger than I am, and I think it has to do with using aloe on my skin."

Vernon Pruitt summarizes his feelings about aloe vera's place in cosmetics this way: "The use of aloe vera in cosmetics has come a long way, but it has a long way to go, both in science and in manufacturing products. We have not seen aloe vera used in all major products where it can be beneficial, but we're getting closer. Years ago major cosmetic companies only put the name 'aloe' on the front label for pizzazz. Today it is not only a popular ingredient, but legitimate scientific studies are causing people to believe that it really is functional in cosmetics."

HEALING THE INSIDE: ARTHRITIS, STOMACH ULCERS, DIABETES, AND MORE 9

Listening to aloe vera believers rattle off a list of the internal problems that it helps to alleviate is almost like listening to faith healers at a revival meeting. Aloe vera juices and gels are used regularly by some people to manage arthritis, stomach ulcers, diabetes, and high blood pressure as well as to boost energy and vitality. Others drink aloe vera occasionally to overcome indigestion, constipation, and diarrhea. Just as with its other uses, however, little scientific research has been conducted on the internal benefits of the plant extracts, so the burden of proof lies in personal testimonials.

ARTHRITIS

Anne Kouba of Rockdale, Texas, drinks a glass of half aloe vera juice and half water and ice every day to help control rheumatoid arthritis in her hands. Although skeptical at first, three months after she began drinking the aloe vera juice she began feeling better. "I'm intelligent enough to know that it may all be in my head, but sometimes when my fingers are real stiff, the juice seems to help lessen the pain," Anne says. "Plus, aloe vera makes me feel cleansed and refreshed. I'm not crazy about the taste, but I got used to it. Now I actually look forward to my daily glass."

When an Olympic athlete from Australia had success using aloe vera to treat sports injuries, she suggested that her grandmother try it as a remedy for arthritis. In a letter to Forever Living, the young woman reported that her grandmother began drinking aloe vera juice four times a day in four-teaspoon doses and applying an aloe vera heat lotion to her hands and neck. She wrote that her grandmother experienced immediate relief from the arthritis in her hands, and "after using one bottle of the juice, she can move her fingers in directions which the arthritis previously had restricted. . . . She also found herself able to turn her head to the right, which she has not been able to do for five years."

In her research on aloe vera, writer Laurie Taylor-Donald found that although many people get immediate relief from arthritis pain, it takes most people up to two months before they feel the effect. Taylor-Donald says that those who report relief from stiffness and pain usually take one or two tablespoons of aloe vera juice two to four times a day.

In a testimonial letter to American Dream International, a man wrote that the arthritis in his hands was so bad that his fingers began to "curl": "I couldn't close my hand or make a fist. There were knots on both elbows the size of golf balls, and I was unable to raise my arms above my shoulders." The man's condition began to change, however, when he began drinking two ounces of aloe vera juice a day. Today, more than five years later, he says that he has no more pain in his hands and that the knots on his elbows have disappeared.

Aloe vera also works on arthritis when it is applied externally. Some aloe users say they feel relief when they rub the gel directly onto the skin over an aching joint or muscle.

Robert H. Davis, Ph.D., professor of physiology at Pennsylvania College of Podiatric Medicine in Philadelphia, recently completed a study of the benefit of aloe vera as a topical application for rheumatoid arthritis. Dr. Davis measured the development and regression of adjuvant arthritis (artificially induced arthritis) in rats treated with aloe vera compared with rats not treated. "Adjuvant arthritis is virtually identical to human rheumatoid arthritis," says Dr. Davis. "The lower limbs of the animals become deformed and the bones are almost completely destroyed."

In his study, the rats were first treated subcutaneously with injections of aloe vera, and he found that the aloe vera helped the arthritis to regress. Then he pasted a poultice of aloe vera, RNA (ribonucleic acid), and vitamin C on the arthritic portion of the rat's body. "I added the vitamin C and RNA because aloe vera is not strong enough by itself to completely eliminate a powerful disease like rheumatoid arthritis," says Dr. Davis. "Aloe vera has great anti-arthritic activity, but I believe the synergistic effects of combining it with vitamin C and RNA make it even more effective."

According to Dr. Davis, RNA redirects the immunological condition in the affected area: "In rheumatoid arthritis, the template (protein mold) in the cytoplasm (the structural RNA) is getting the wrong information from the cell nucleus. The RNA in this treatment goes into the cell and enables the nucleus to provide the correct information."

The aloe vera/vitamin C/RNA treatment returned the arthritic areas of the rats' bodies to normal. Dr. Davis says this treatment was even more effective than the aloe vera injections. In many cases it prevented the arthritis from developing, and if arthritis did develop, the improvement was quicker and greater with the combined treatment method.

STOMACH DISORDERS

For years North and Central American Indians have used aloe vera juice as a tonic to aid in digestion and elimination and to treat ulcers. The ethnopharmacological archives at Pan American University in Edinburg, Texas, contain more than 3,000 cases of home remedies—many involving the use of aloe vera to treat stomach problems, according to Robert Trotter II, director for research and development.

"One unusual method I remember for treating ulcers involved swallowing a one-inch long cut of the leaf every morning," says Dr. Trotter. "An ulcer is a wound that is somewhat similar to a burn, so used that way, the aloe vera may promote the type of healing it does with burns. But I wouldn't advise it."

Today, people caution against ingesting the yellow sap because of its powerful laxative properties. "It's not a healthy practice to drink a laxative every day," says Ray Henry, former senior vice president and technical director of Aloe Laboratories of Texas, Inc., in Harlingen. "The laxative in it is a gastric irritant."

Aloe vera seems to have homeostatic properties. Whereas some people use it to control constipation, others use it to control diarrhea.

Bill McAnalley, former vice president and research director of Carrington Laboratories in Dallas, says he has hundreds of reports from people who have cured various chronic bowel problems and ulcers by drinking aloe vera. "We received one letter from a businessman who had stomach ulcers for years," he recalls. "The doctors finally told him to go somewhere to get away from his business. He went down to the Rio Grande Valley, and while there someone told him about aloe vera. He was skeptical, but figured he had nothing to lose. He began drinking aloe vera daily and started feeling much better. He hasn't had any problems in five years."

According to McAnalley, another Carrington Laboratories customer is a public speaker who had had two operations for stomach problems before he began drinking aloe vera. "As long as he drinks aloe vera juice, he doesn't have any problems. The problem is that some people say their friends tease them about drinking aloe vera, so they quit using it and their stomach problems return. Some of our customers say they have stopped drinking the juice several times, but they always go back to it."

Art Benson, a Carrington Laboratories distributor from North Hollywood, California, became interested in aloe vera when his sister-in-law was cured of bleeding ulcers. "She was scheduled for surgery, but the night before the operation her daughter called from Texas with some family problems," recalls Benson. "She went to Dallas to help out and she drank Carrington Laboratories' Cellogel the whole two weeks she was there. When she returned to California, she went to her doctor for an X-ray, and nothing showed up. The doctor didn't believe it and took another set of X-rays. He wanted to know what she had used and he ended up buying $250 worth of the product."

Four to eight ounces of aloe vera juice a day over the last

six years are what Don Thompson, president of American Dream International, Inc., in Visalia, California, credits for his healed stomach. "I used to have an ulcerated stomach and a hiatal hernia; I couldn't eat spicy foods. Now I can eat any type of food I want without any side effects, not even heartburn." Thompson believes that room-temperature aloe works faster in the stomach: "The stomach absorbs it better when it's not cold."

A woman from Crystal Springs, Mississippi, who is a distributor for American Dream International says she had had ulcers eight times and was ready to have part of her stomach surgically removed when her mother-in-law introduced her to aloe vera juice. "I had used aloe vera for scratches and burns, and it was the fastest healing thing I ever saw," says sixty-year-old Dottie Wilson. "I didn't know that people drank aloe vera, so I tried it. It had a somewhat unpleasant flavor, but it cured the ulcer."

Bill Coats, R.Ph., of Coats Aloe International, believes that aloe vera does a lot of the same things drugs do but without the side effects. "One commonly used ulcer drug is great to treat ulcers, but it can cause impotency," says Coats. "I spoke to one doctor who says he has seen ulcers healed in thirty days by using a combination of aloe vera drink, an ulcer diet, and an antacid."

According to McAnalley, people who go from a quality product to one with less aloe in it often find that their problems return. "People with stomach problems seem to get relief by drinking three to four ounces of our juice a day," he says. "It's best not to drink it all at one time but to take it an ounce or so at a time, so aloe vera can be kept in the stomach throughout the day.

Suzanne Jackson of San Diego doesn't drink aloe vera regularly but takes it when needed for heartburn and indigestion. "It knocks it out in five minutes," she says.

James Fulton, M.D., a dermatologist from Newport Beach, California, uses aloe vera gel in his practice to treat acne, and he says he drinks the juice as needed to relieve gastritis from drinking too much coffee.

In 1985 a scientific study on the effects of aloe vera on the gastrointestinal tract was performed by Jeffrey S. Bland, Ph.D., president of Healthcomm, Inc., in Gig Harbor, Washington. Dr. Bland studied the effects of aloe vera on the gastrointestinal tract of ten healthy individuals. In the article "Effect of Orally Consumed Aloe Vera Juice on Gastrointestinal Function In Normal Humans" (published in *Preventive Medicine,* March/April 1985), Dr. Bland confirmed that aloe vera juice is well tolerated and does not produce any overt gastrointestinal side effects.

A product that contains significant quantities of yellow sap, however, may cause gastric problems for some individuals. Aloe vera product manufacturers indicate that 50 to 300 parts of yellow sap per million is a safe ratio. Some companies believe that small amounts of aloin in an aloe vera drink improve the value of aloe vera because it helps move waste through the intestinal tract.

Among other things, Dr. Bland's study showed that aloe vera improves bowel motility, reduces the indication of protein putrefaction in the colon, and improves colonic bacterial function. The researcher says that more studies remain to be done on the impact of aloe vera on patients with gastrointestinal problems, such as colitis and inflammatory bowel disease.

CONTROLLING BLOOD PRESSURE, DIABETES, AND OTHER PROBLEMS

"We hear a lot of stories about why people use aloe vera, and high blood pressure is one reason we hear repeatedly," says Ray Henry. "People say, 'I had high blood pressure but since I've been drinking aloe vera, the doctor has reduced the amount of medication I take.'"

Bill Coats of Coats Aloe International agrees that aloe vera juice lowers blood pressure. "I used to be on medication to treat high blood pressure," he says, "but the medication made me drowsy. My salespeople told me that aloe vera works to treat high blood pressure. At that time I was only taking about an ounce of aloe vera a day. I increased that to six ounces a day and within a short period of time, my blood pressure was down to normal. It has stayed at about 120/80 for 10 years, but if I don't take aloe vera, it shoots back up to about 150/100."

Lou Mossbauer, distributor of aloe vera products and a diabetic, claims that aloe vera juice helped to make his life insulin-free: "It took about nine months, but I haven't had to take insulin for years. One of my customers also stopped taking insulin after drinking aloe vera for a year."

For distributor Art Benson, aloe vera helped cure not only his diabetes but a host of other health conditions. "I had suffered two heart attacks; had acute bronchitis, gout, uremic poisoning, and kidney stones; and was receiving cortisone shots for bursitis and arthritis," says Benson. "My brother sent me some aloe vera for my fifty-eighth birthday. In three months I was off insulin, and the gout, kidney stones, and arthritis all disappeared."

Barbara Hetrick of El Cajon, California, says she had been

suffering from thrombosis (inflammation of veins in the legs) and was prone to getting blood clots. After taking aloe vera juice she never had the problem again.

Bill Coats relates the story of a woman from St. Louis who had multiple sclerosis and could walk only with crutches. "Six days before one of the Forever Living distributors' meetings she purchased some gel and drink," says Coats. "When the meeting day arrived, she walked to the meeting without crutches. The aloe vera drink took away the soreness and inflammation in her joints, which had made it so painful for her to walk."

A change to vegetarian diet that included daily supplements of aloe vera juice is what Mary Wilson of Carson City, Nevada, credits for helping to rid her body of tumors. "I was very sick and the doctors wanted to amputate my leg, but I wouldn't let them," says Wilson. "I changed my diet and read everything I could about aloe vera. I started drinking the juice daily and my health turned around because I had the proper amino acid, carbohydrate and protein balance in my system. My body is free of tumors and I saved my leg. I had to wear a brace and use crutches for a year, but I learned to walk again."

One novel study by the Spokane Veterans Outreach Center in Spokane, Washington, treated individuals suffering from drug and alcohol abuse with Forever Living Products, including aloe vera juice, a diet supplement, and bee pollen. A report describing the study said that the aloe vera was used to cleanse the body of toxins. The other products were used to increase metabolism, supplement nutrition, increase energy, and assist in the rebuilding of the body's immune system. The results indicated that of the fifty people treated, the recovery process was hastened in the twenty-five who used the prescribed products. Whether or not this study can be duplicated in an independent scientific study remains to be seen.

A General Health Drink

While many people drink aloe to overcome an illness, some drink a daily dose as a way to prevent illness because they believe that aloe vera is a natural detoxifier. Because it has only eight calories per ounce, aloe vera juice is also a non-fattening addition to a diet, like many other vegetable juices.

Some people report that they have more energy and more vitality when they drink aloe vera juice. "It gives you a tremendous amount of energy," says Lou Mossbauer, an aloe vera distributor in San Diego. "In fact, if you drink too much of it in the evening, you'll wake up at two or three o'clock in the morning."

Mossbauer believes that the body dictates how much aloe vera a person needs. "My grandson and his friend drink aloe vera juice an hour before they go surfing. They claim that their energy peaks about an hour later when they are out on the waves."

Don Thompson says that since he began drinking aloe vera six years ago, he has not suffered from any major illness and neither have his children. "It's a colon cleanser," he says. "We keep a gallon of aloe vera juice sitting on the kitchen counter because we feel it's a preventive medicine and a natural remedy."

ALOE VERA
FIGHTS TOOTH AND
GUM DECAY

10

People frequently associate aloe vera with the treatment of burns, scrapes, and ulcers, but how many people—even avid aloe vera users—think of using aloe vera on the teeth and gums? For dentist Bill Wolfe, from Albuquerque, New Mexico, that's the first thing that comes to mind when he's asked about the plant.

When Dr. Wolfe became interested in using aloe vera in his dental practice, he was disappointed to find how little scientific research had been done on the subject. While performing his own research, he came across the studies of one of his former college professors, the late Eugene R. Zimmermann, M.A., D.D.S., professor of pathology at Baylor College of Dentistry, in Dallas, Texas.

Dr. Zimmermann had compared aloe vera with two other anti-inflammatory drugs, indomethacin and prednisolone (as reported in the January, 1969 issue of *Oral Surgery, Oral Medicine and Oral Pathology*). He found aloe vera to be just as effective as the two anti-inflammatory drugs and with an added

94

benefit—aloe vera didn't harm the tissue culture cells, whereas prednisolone and indomethacin were toxic to the tissues over a period of time.

Intrigued by Dr. Zimmermann's findings, Dr. Wolfe offered to fund further studies on aloe vera's usefulness in fighting dental plaque and in stimulating healing after surgery. "Dr. Zimmermann was well-known for his studies on fluoride and dental fluorosis (excessive fluoride)," says Dr. Wolfe. After months of research, Dr. Zimmermann tested and developed a specific aloe vera gel to be used in dentistry.

"Our lab tests showed that the Aloe Vera Oral Gel was effective as a bacteriocidal or bacteriostatic agent against five strains of a microorganism important to tooth decay," said Dr. Zimmermann. "It was also found to be non-toxic to one line of tissue culture cells." Dr. Wolfe adds, "That means that after one week of using the gel, patients look as though they've had three weeks of healing time."

Dr. Wolfe now uses Aloe Vera Oral Gel in several ways in his dental practice. When fitting new dentures he applies the gel directly to the dentures. "The dentures act like a bandage to hold the aloe vera next to the gums to help them heal," explains Dr. Wolfe. "The average period of time to wait to remove stitches after extracting teeth for immediate dentures is three days. When we use aloe vera, we can remove the stitches the following day. Aloe vera is an anti-inflammatory, with a steroid-like aspect; and it numbs while it heals," says Dr. Wolfe. "I have found that when aloe vera is used many patients don't need to take any pain medication after surgery."

Dr. Wolfe also recommends using Aloe Vera Oral Gel for denture patients with sore mouths. He also uses the gel to reduce irritation and inflammation around exposed roots and sore gums often caused by temporary crowns.

Dr. Wolfe decided to carry the research on aloe vera a step further to develop an aloe vera toothpaste: "Many of my patients who used the gel to reduce inflammation after a tooth extraction, denture delivery, or oral surgery were using the gel at home as a toothpaste, but they disliked the bitter taste. After two years of research, Dr. Zimmermann developed a formula for a toothpaste that is not only pleasant tasting but has the same bactericidal effects as the Aloe Vera Oral Gel."

The toothpaste, named Aloe-Dent, is produced and distributed by Pepperdent, the same company in Orlando, Florida, that markets the Aloe Vera Oral Gel to dentists and dental laboratories. "Most toothpastes include dyes, sugars, and fluoride, as well as baking soda and salt as an abrasive," says Dr. Wolfe. "Aloe-Dent has no artificial colors or fluoride. It has a minimum amount of mint flavoring and is sweetened with Nutrasweet, which is made of two amino acids. Unlike other toothpastes, Aloe-Dent will not only clean the teeth but heal the gums as well."

Dr. Zimmermann believed that aloe vera could be useful for other problems with the teeth and mouth, such as mouth ulcers caused by mental stress and food allergies.

Another dentist who believes in aloe vera is Rick Chavez, D.D.S., of Seattle, Washington. "I use a lubricant when I perform a root canal so that the tooth material doesn't pack down at the end of the root," he explains. "The idea of a root canal is to clean the tooth down to about three-quarters of a millimeter from the end of the root. If you keep it lubricated, the tooth material will stay in suspension. A variety of materials can be used for this, even water, but I find that aloe vera works best."

Dr. Chavez also finds aloe vera to be useful in oral surgery: "After an extraction, I place some aloe vera on a piece of gauze and have the patient bite down. This helps ease the pain and aids in healing. My uncle experienced this first-hand," Dr. Chavez continues. "After his wisdom tooth was removed, he placed the inside of an aloe vera leaf on his gum and the pain immediately subsided."

In emergency situations with bone and gum problems, Dr. Chavez rubs aloe vera in and under the gum to cleanse and soothe the area until the patient can see a periodontist. "I use aloe vera because it works, not because I'm making any money off of it," Dr. Chavez explains. "It works for me but I'm not saying it will work for everyone. It doesn't do any harm and I've seen it do some good."

So has Art Benson of North Hollywood, California, who claims that aloe vera toothpaste stops dental decay and gingivitis.

It may not be common in dentistry yet, but if people like Dr. Wolfe have their way, more and more dentists will begin treating their patients with aloe vera.

TREATING SPORTS INJURIES WITH ALOE VERA

11

In recent years aloe vera has begun to muscle its way onto the sports scene, and a wide spectrum of athletes, from weekend joggers to professional football stars, are beginning to appreciate the benefits it has to offer—though some athletes might not be interested in aloe vera's softening effects on their skin. Ozzie Smith, shortstop for the St. Louis Cardinals, softens the pocket of his baseball glove by rubbing it with aloe vera lotion in combination with shaving cream and leather balm.

Aloe vera is used to treat a variety of sports injuries. It reduces inflammation of strained muscles, soothes turf burns, and helps heal blisters. As head athletic trainer at the University of Texas in Austin, Spanky Stephens, co-author of *Healing Winners,* uses aloe vera for conditions such as muscle sprains, cramps, blisters, sunburn, turf burns, minor aches and pains, and major injuries. Stephens relies on aloe vera products because of their ability to penetrate quickly into the skin. "Aloe vera helps to increase cell healing time and speeds up cell reproduction to heal injured tissue," he says. "We've had many instances in which we've used it on an injured player who, with the traditional treatment, wouldn't have been able to play for weeks, but by using the aloe vera is out on the field the following week."

Stephens also uses aloe vera creams to "piggyback" other substances into the skin tissue. He often mixes aloe vera cream with an aspirin-based methyl salicylate product. Placed on the injury, the aloe vera quickly absorbs into the tissue, taking the other products with it and speeding up the healing process.

"Aloe is so versatile," Stephens points out. "It can be used on all parts of the body without worrying about burning or irritation. And you can apply it as often as you like."

While Stephens finds aloe vera useful in all sports—football, basketball, tennis, track and field, golf, swimming, and diving—he says it's especially helpful with turf burns. "With most products, turf burns leave scars, but when we use aloe vera we see almost no scarring at all."

One method of application that Stephens currently uses is to freeze the aloe vera juice, then massage it into the body. "The ice closes down the capillaries for surface bleeding and tissue bleeding, and the aloe penetrates into the tissue and helps with pain. When we use this treatment in conjunction with an aspirin-based product, we receive double the effectiveness."

Stephens uses Forever Living Products, including Aloe Vera Activator, Aloe Lotion, and Aloe Heat Lotion. "The Aloe Heat Lotion is used for athletes with sore hands and feet, or those who have muscle aches and pains," he says. "It doesn't get real hot, but you can feel heat penetrate into the system."

In an article printed in a Forever Living Products brochure, gold medal gymnast Kurt Thomas discusses how he used Aloe Heat Lotion to heal his chapped, cracked hands after hours of practicing and performing.

Other world-class athletes have also used aloe vera products. According to Stephens, aloe vera was first used by the U.S. Olympic Committee at the 1976 Montreal Games. "When you are working with a large group of athletes, it's easier if you can reduce the number of products you use and heal them just as fast with one product—aloe vera. It's a great product because it does so many things."

Regarding the controversy about the curative powers of aloe vera, Stephens says, "The fact that there is a folklore surrounding aloe vera makes some people doubtful of the claims. One reason some people may not think aloe vera works is because they don't know how to apply it. If you had pneumonia and took one penicillin capsule, that wouldn't cure the problem. The same is true with aloe vera. If you put aloe vera on an injury just one time it won't be effective. It must be applied properly and thoroughly."

As assistant trainer for the Dallas Cowboys football team for the past fifteen years, Ken Locker has seen a variety of sports injuries. In the beginning he was doubtful that aloe vera could do all the things people said it could. As he says, "Some people claim it will cure anything from cancer to athlete's foot, and that's a pretty broad spectrum."

Locker points out that in most medical journals in the United States, there is one specific medication to treat one specific form of pathology. "For arthritis you use an anti-inflammatory or pain medication, for acid indigestion an antacid is usually prescribed, and for athlete's foot you use an antifungal medication," he says. "No one believes that one medication can cure all three ailments."

Locker says he was initially amazed that something derived from a plant could be so effective, but he has discovered that the more you use aloe vera, the more it works. "You either accept the success of the treatment as luck or you become convinced that aloe vera can aid the body's healing mechanisms."

Locker has been using aloe for more than twelve years to treat a variety of ailments, including first-degree sprained ankles, sprained knees, turf burns, sunburn, and fungus problems such as athlete's foot. "It has a great application for acute injuries and chronic symptoms that occur in athletics," he says.

Locker uses Forever Living Products—the juice for digestive purposes and the Activator and Gelly to saturate gauze and bandages that will be applied to wounds and acute injuries. "For sunburn and to soothe skin problems and irritations, I like Aloe Vera Lotion. And to treat tendinitis, sprains, and strains, I rely on Aloe Heat Lotion made with eucalyptus oil, which serves as a counter-irritant," he says. "For the more acute injuries, I use an aloe vera ice pack to wrap around the injured part."

With the stampede of after-work joggers that has emerged during the last several years, some of the most common sports injuries today are running-related. According to *Runners World,* runners of all ages and abilities sustain, on the average, at least one injury per year. That figure increases dramatically for runners over the age of thirty who run more than thirty miles a week. The foot, ankle, knee, shin, and muscles of the upper leg are the most susceptible because they are subjected to the greatest amount of strain.

Brooks Johnson, director of track and field in the Department of Athletics at Stanford University, finds aloe vera helpful in treating just those types of injuries. Johnson had heard about people with critical health problems who had been helped by aloe vera and decided to try using it on his runners. He was so pleased with the results that he has been using aloe vera to treat a variety of sports injuries for the past three years.

Foxfield Products of Sacramento, California, supplies Johnson with the aloe vera products he uses, which include aloe vera juice and gel, a heat rub that can be used topically, and an aloe vera–based spray that relieves rashes, "jock itch," and athlete's foot, and helps heal abrasions.

When one of Johnson's runners is injured, he uses aloe vera to reduce inflammation. "It's especially good for aspirin-sensitive athletes because it can be rubbed on topically with aspirin, thereby bypassing the stomach and avoiding upset," he says. "For those who are aspirin-tolerant, the penetrating properties of aloe vera help take the aspirin right into the bloodstream. And since it's not diluted it works much faster."

Aloe vera has also proved to be an effective food supplement for Johnson's distance runners, who mix it with other juices to get an energy boost.

In their book *Healing Winners,* Bill Coats and Spanky Stephens offer suggestions on treating sports injuries at home with aloe vera products. The authors, however, stress that the treatments they recommend should not supersede a visit to a physician or other qualified professional. In general, they suggest that aloe vera products can be used to treat sports injuries in the following ways (the specific products the authors suggest are listed in parentheses and are produced by Forever Living Products):

Blisters: After cleansing the blister, soak it in aloe vera juice (Stabilized Aloe Activator) for about five minutes to relieve pain and fight bacteria. Then cut a small hole in the bottom of the blister. Using a cotton swab, apply aloe vera gel (Aloe Vera Gelly) into the hole to reduce infection and protect the blister. Finally, expose the blistered area to air to hasten healing.

Sprains: To supplement soaking the sprained area in ice, the authors suggest using an ice rub made of frozen aloe vera juice (Aloe Activator) to reduce swelling and relieve pain. If a reinforcing wrap is needed, they suggest seeing a professional sports trainer or physician.

Muscle strains: To allow the muscle to heal properly, Stephens and Coats caution the athlete not to resume activity until the muscle is pain-free and complete movement is restored. If the muscle is swollen, they suggest using a cold pack of ice made with aloe vera and a gentle massage with an aloe vera lotion (Aloe Lotion). After forty-eight hours the ice packs may be alternated with hot whirlpool soakings and intermittent applications of an aloe vera heat rub (Aloe Heat Lotion) to reduce swelling and speed recovery.

Turf burns and other lesions: Cleanse the area with a pharmaceutical cleanser, such as Phisohex or Betadine solutions. Apply hydrogen peroxide to the area and cover with a dressing soaked with aloe vera gel (Stabilized Aloe Vera Gelly). Replace the dressing daily to guard against infection.

VETERINARY USES 12

After hearing about the many ways aloe vera heals injuries and illnesses, some people credit the placebo effect: the healing that takes place is more psychological than physiological. That may be true in some instances, but how then can the testimonials about animals who have been healed by aloe vera be explained?

An Olympic athlete from Australia, who had used Forever Living Products to treat sports injuries, said that she recommended that her grandfather use aloe vera to help heal rat bites suffered by his prize-winning roosters. Officials at the local agricultural department had suggested using Vaseline, but the sores had failed to heal. In a letter to Forever Living Products, the woman said that she and her grandfather treated half of the roosters with Aloe Activator and the other half with Vaseline. She also squirted aloe vera juice down the throats of the group she was treating with aloe vera.

Within twenty-four hours, those treated with aloe vera had started to heal while the others had worsened. They began treat-

ing the whole group with aloe vera and within three days the
sores had healed completely. In fact, she reported, the birds were
healthier than they had ever been.

Skin care hygienist Julie Russell, from Escondido, California, is an avid fan of aloe vera. Once, she fed some boiled aloe
vera juice to a friend's dog, and the animal's arthritis was greatly
alleviated. "It really works," she insists.

When Dottie Wilson of Crystal Springs, Mississippi, raised
Chihuahuas, she used the gel directly from the plant to treat
their wounds.

Bill Coats, of Coats Aloe International is the author of *Crea-
tures in Our Care,* which describes how aloe vera can be helpful
to animals. "It does wonders for the swelling in horses' legs,"
Coats says. "Trainers saturate a cotton pad with aloe vera juice
and wrap it around the horse's leg. Then they place plastic wrap
around the pad so the juice won't evaporate, and a stretch bandage over that. After twenty-four hours, the swelling is gone."

Coats also believes aloe vera is effective when added to an
animal's food. A man he knew in California raised racing pigeons, but the pigeons had never been in the top 100 in any
race. "He added aloe vera to their food and drink, and in the
next major race his birds took second, tenth, and twentieth
places. It may have been coincidence, but it certainly paid off."

As a racehorse owner, Coats feels that horses also benefit
when aloe vera is added to their food. "Nothing is too good for
my racehorses," he says. "They get hot meals, a bath every
day, and aloe vera in their feed. The aloe vera helps to break
down proteins, fats, and starches, which makes the horses uti-
lize their food better."

Some people use aloe vera to combat their pets' fleas. "A

customer's dogs had been scratching themselves to death from fleas," says Lou Mossbauer, an aloe vera distributor from San Diego. "She put aloe vera gel on the flea-bitten areas and added aloe vera juice to their drinking water. Not only are her dogs free of fleas, but they love water with aloe in it."

In his book *The Aloe Vera Handbook,* Max B. Skousen, Director of Aloe Vera Research Institute, points out that animals often suffer from digestive disorders, arthritis, and other internal ailments. He suggests adding aloe vera to their food on a regular basis for the same soothing and healing benefits that it has on humans. He also points out that aloe vera is effective as a topical treatment to help heal wounds and infections in animals.

The therapeutic uses of a portion of aloe's carbohydrate materials, (e.g. acemannan) within the animal kingdom is seen in the successful treatment of Marek's disease, a highly infectious and deadly virus that affects poultry and can be devastating to a poultry farmer. The addition of acemannan to the vaccine significantly enhanced its effectiveness. Acemannan has also been successfully added to vaccines that are effectively treating cat leukemia and dog viruses.

WHAT'S NEXT? 13

In 1988, Carrington Laboratories identified and patented acemannan, a complex polysaccharide and carbohydrate derivative that is considered by them to be the major therapeutically active ingredient in aloe vera gel. They are also responsible for devising a method of ensuring its stability and purity. By doing so, the company opened the way for further studies on its therapeutic activities. Because acemannan is so stable, it does not metabolize until it reaches the target cell. It interacts with the immune system and thus acts as an immunomodulator, that is, a compound that stimulates immune cell function and cytosine synthesis. Therefore, its potential for anti-viral and anti-inflammatory abilities may make it useful in the treatment of infectious diseases.

Part of the excitement surrounding the applications of aloe-derived materials is that biotech companies around the world are attempting to produce a variety of carbohydrate-based drugs. The reason is that carbohydrates are no longer considered merely an energy source for intracellular metabolism. Scientists have discovered that carbohydrates can be potentially useful in a wide range of substances that can interact with and fight diseases within the immune system for both animals and humans. Although some may call this approach a panacea, the research on aloe derivatives being conducted by biotech firms and aloe scientists has opened the door to the development of new aloe products with significant healing results.

CROSSING THE THRESHOLD INTO MAINSTREAM MEDICINE

In the last few years, a variety of effective and popular products have been successfully used by health care professionals. For example, clinicians, surgeons, and radiation oncologists across the country are using aloe-based ointments in wound dressings. These types of products have been found to accelerate the healing of wounds and also to enhance the quality of healing in terms of cosmetic acceptability and wound integrity. They are most effective in the care of ulcers, wounds, burns, and other skin-related ailments.

WHAT THE FUTURE HOLDS

The most significant areas of growth and interest within the aloe industry, from a commercial as well as a scientific perspective, are these:

1. An increase in the standards being placed on the industry, which will further promote the natural and scientifically based healing abilities of aloe. Efforts are being made by industry leaders to focus on manufacturing, quality assurance, and process development functions. At the same time, new deriva-

tives of acemannan-like aloe substances will be tested for superior efficacy in different applications. Moreover, several analytical methods for the standardization of raw aloe vera gel and the truly active aloe content in liquid commercial products are being developed in several laboratories. These new assays will help the aloe industry by creating a level playing field for aloe producers, identifying fraudulent companies and giving regulatory agencies a basis for prosecuting violators.

2. Further industry standards for establishing active aloe in products, which will improve industry credibility and help cull out the opportunists from the dedicated professionals.

3. Future research, including intensive research of aloe substances at a molecular level. According to Dr. Winters, there will also be more emphasis on the creation of synthetic products from aloe substances that may have the ability to act as highly potent anti-tumor and anti-viral drugs.

4. Further FDA approval of new drugs and products to help in the treatment of cancer and infectious diseases such as AIDS. Dr. Winters is also conducting research that shows the positive effect of using aloe in relation to neural cell functions. According to Dr. Winters, a new paper being published in the scientific literature describes for the first time the effects of aloe substances on neuron-like cells. Further research may show that aloe can help with neural illnesses such as cerebral palsy, multiple sclerosis, and Alzheimer's disease.

International scientifically validated research studies, coupled with stringent enforcement of FDA labeling laws, are helping the aloe industry to obtain and maintain credibility and to make new discoveries about effective applications of the natural healing powers of aloe. As we face the twenty-first century, it is anticipated that more studies will prove that aloe truly is a pharmacy in a plant. Aloe may come to be used in treating some of the world's most devastating illnesses and, at the same time, offer continued relief of some of our most common aches and pains.

APPENDIX A

DEFINITIONS

Acemannan A complex carbohydrate considered to be one of many active ingredients found in aloe.

Raw Aloe Vera Gel Naturally occurring, unprocessed, undiluted parenchymal tissue obtained from the decorticated leaves of *Aloe barbadensis* Miller (*Aloe vera* Line), to which no other material has been added.

Aloe Vera Gel Naturally occurring, processed, undiluted parenchymal tissue obtained from the decorticated leaves of *Aloe barbadensis* Miller.

100 Percent Aloe Vera Processed, preserved liquid derived from parenchymal tissue obtained from the decorticated leaves of *Aloe barbadensis* Miller (*Aloe vera* Line) containing not more than 50 ppm aloin and defined by a value of 1,000 using the reporting procedure adopted by the NASC.

Whole Aloe Vera Gel Aloe Vera Gel, which contains a minimum of 50 percent of the natural pulp found in Raw Aloe Vera Gel.

Aloe Vera Latex The bitter yellow liquid contained in the pericyclic tubules of the rind of *Aloe barbadensis* Miller; the principal constituent of which is aloin.

Whole Leaf Aloe Vera Whole leaf of the *Aloe barbadensis* Miller, including the rind and internal portions of the plant.

Aloe USP The dried latex of the leaves of *Aloe barbadensis* Miller (*Aloe vera* Line), known in commerce as Curaçao Aloe or Aloe Ferox Miller and hybrids of this species, with *Aloe africana* Miller and *Aloe spicata* Baker, known in commerce as Cape Aloe (Liliaceae).

Aloe Vera Oil The lipid protein obtained from the leaves of *Aloe barbadensis* Miller by various solvent extraction processes.

Stabilized Aloe Vera Gel Synonymous with the term Aloe Vera Gel.

Aloe Vera Pulp The parenchymal tissue and fiber derived from Raw Aloe Vera.

Aloe Vera Concentrate Aloe Vera Gel, from which natural water has been mechanically removed and which would have a value of 1,500 minimum using the reporting procedure adopted by the NASC.

Reconstituted Aloe Vera Gel Aloe vera concentrate, to which an appropriate amount of water has been added to achieve a concentration that is equivalent to 100 percent aloe vera as defined above.

Aloe Vera Gel, Spray Dried Aqueous derivative of the leaf of *Aloe barbadensis* Miller, which has been spray dried on a suitable matrix.

Reconstituted Aloe Vera Gel, Spray Dried Aloe Vera Gel Spray Dried, to which an appropriate amount of water has been added to achieve concentration that is equivalent to 100 percent Aloe Vera as defined above.

Aloe Vera Gel, Freeze Dried Aloe Vera Gel that has been freeze dried with or without a matrix.

Reconstituted Aloe Vera Gel, Freeze Dried Aloe Vera Gel Freeze Dried, to which an appropriate amount of water has been added to achieve a concentration that is equivalent to 100 percent Aloe Vera as defined above.

Aloe Vera Juice An ingestible product containing a minimum of 50 percent Aloe Vera Gel, as defined by the reporting procedure adopted by the NASC.

Aloe Vera Drink An ingestible product containing less than 50 percent and more than 10 percent of Aloe Vera Gel, as defined by the reporting procedure adopted by the NASC.

Aloe Vera Extract A dilution of *Aloe barbadensis* Miller with water or other suitable solvents that contains less than 10 percent Aloe Vera, as defined by the reporting procedure adopted by the NASC, and is suitable for ingestion or topical use.

(Reprinted with permission from the National Aloe Science Council.)

Appendix

Useful Addresses

If you are interested in learning more about the many aloe vera products available, the following companies can provide more information:

Chesebrough Ponds
   800 Sylvan Avenue
   Englewood Cliffs, NJ 07632
   (800) 743-8640
   retail sales only

Forever Living Products
   P.O. Box 29041
   Phoenix, AZ 85038
   (602) 968-3999
   brochure available

Fruit of the Earth, Inc.
   P.O. Box 727
   Bensonville, IL 60106
   (312) 766-5400
   retail only (800) 527-7731

General Nutrition, Inc.
   Mail Order Division
   921 Penn Ave.
   Pittsburgh, PA 15222
   (412) 288-4600
   mail-order catalog

Key West Aloe
   524 Front St.
   Key West, FL 33040
   mail-order catalog
   (305) 294-5592
   (800) 445-2563

Rachel Perry Cosmetics
   9111 Mason Ave.
   Chatsworth, CA 91311
   (818) 888-5881
   brochure available

BIBLIOGRAPHIC NOTES

Ace, Edith L. *Healing With Aloe Vera: The Poor Man's Pharmacy.* Pataskala, OH: Ace Publications, 1979.

"Add Zest to Daily Living." Hilltop Gardens, Lyford, TX.

"Aloe: Super Summer Soother." *Harper's Bazaar,* July 1982, p. 60.

"Aloe Vera Council Defends Its Practices, Product." *FDA Consumer,* November 1981, p. 29.

Aloe Vera Letters: True Healing Experiences. Denver, CO: Royal Publications, 1983.

"Aloe Verified." *Organic Gardening & Farming,* August 1981, p. 46.

The Amazing Ancient to Modern Useful Plant Aloe Vera, Lemon Grove, CA: Prevo Publications, 1984.

Ayensu, Edward S. "A Worldwide Role for the Healing Powers of Plants." *Smithsonian,* 12 November 1981, p. 87.

Banks, David H. *Nature's Genie: Aloe Vera.* Florence, OR: West Publishers, 1981.

"Beneficient Botanicals: Plant Extracts for Cosmetic and Medicinal Purposes." *New York Times Magazine,* 22 February 1981, p. 82.

BioSearch Laboratories, Inc. "Analysis No. L368—Streptococcus Mutans." Arlington, TX, January 1980.

Bland, Jeffrey S., Ph.D. "Effect of Orally Consumed Aloe Vera Juice on Gastrointestinal Function in Normal Humans." *Preventive Medicine*, March/April 1985.

Blumenthal, Deborah. "The Facts Behind the Aloe Mystique." *New York Times Sunday Magazine*, 6 September 1981, p. 32.

Bonk, Thomas. "Ozzie: Cardinal Shortstop Sets the Standard for Glove Work." *Los Angeles Times*, part III, 23 July 1985.

Brasher, James W., Collings, C. K., and Zimmermann, E. R. "The Effects of Prednisolone, Indomethacin, and Aloe Vera Gel on Tissue Culture Cells." *Oral Surgery, Oral Medicine and Oral Pathology*, 27 (1), 1969, pp. 122–28.

Burns, Frank S. "Substance Abuse and the Use of Forever Living Products During the Early Stages of the Recovery Process." Spokane, WA: Spokane Veterans Outreach Center.

Byers, Theodore E. "Yes, But How Safe?" *Drug and Cosmetic Industry*, September 1984, p. 16.

Carrington Laboratories. "The Logical and Biological Bases for Aloe Vera Gel Properties." Carrington Laboratories, Irving, TX.

Carrington Laboratories. "Physician Experience Report with AVA Topical Stabilized Aloe Gel Products." Carrington Laboratories, Irving, TX.

Cera, L. M., Heggers, J. P., Robson, M. C., and Hagstrom, W. J. "The Therapeutic Efficacy of Aloe Vera Cream (Dermaide Aloe) in Thermal Injuries: Two Case Reports." *Journal of the American Animal Hospital Association*, 16 (September/October), 1980, p. 768.

Chew, Ernest B. "Aloe There." *San Diego Home and Garden*, January 1985, p. 86.

Coats, Bill C., R.Ph. *The Silent Healer: A Modern Study of Aloe Vera*. Garland, TX: Coats, 1979.

Coats, Bill C., R.Ph., and Stephens, Spanky. *Healing Winners: Treating Athletic Injuries with Aloe Vera*. Garland, TX: Coats, 1982.

Duke, J. A. "Overview of Aloe Barbadensis." Economic Botany Laboratory (Building 265, BARC-East), Beltsville, MD.

Encyclopedia Britannica. Subheading Micropedia 15th ed. "Aloe Vera." Chicago: Encyclopedia Britannica, 1974, p. 268.

"Facts and Fancies About Aloe Vera." *Glamour,* December 1979, p. 140.

Fenly, Leigh. "Doctor's ABC of Nutrition." *San Diego Union,* section C, 11 March 1985, p. 1.

Fitch, Charles Marden. "Aloe. The House Plant That Heals." *Flower and Garden,* October/November 1982, p. 34.

The Forever Enterprize. (Nos. 4, 5, and 6) Magazine for Forever Living Distributors, Phoenix, AZ (no dates).

Fox, Arnold. "Aloe Vera and B_{12}—An Important Discovery." *Total Health,* 5 (4), 1983, p. 48.

Gjerstad, Gunnar, and Riner, T. D. "Current Status of Aloe as a Cure-All." *American Journal of Pharmacy,* March/April 1968, p. 58.

Gottlieb, Karen. *Aloe Vera Heals.* Denver, CO: Royal Publications, Inc., 1980.

Halpin, Anne. "Six Useful Plants for Indoor Gardens." *Organic Gardening and Farming,* November, 1980, p. 69.

Hecht, Annabel. "The Overselling of Aloe Vera." *FDA Consumer,* July/August 1981, p. 27.

Heggers, J. P., Pineless, G. R., and Robson, M. C. "Dermaide Aloe/Aloe Vera Gel: Comparison of the Antimicrobial Effects." *Journal of Amercan Medical Technology,* 41, 1979, p. 293.

Heinerman, John. *Aloe Vera, Jojoba and Yucca.* New Canaan, CT: Keats Publishing, Inc., 1982.

Henry, Ray. "An Updated Review of Aloe Vera." *Cosmetics & Toiletries,* 94 (June), 1979, p. 42.

Hermittee, Raoul. "Aloe Vera Literature Review." Phytec Laboratories, National Aloe Science Council, McLean, VA.

"How To Grow Aloe Vera, the First Aid Plant." *Glamour,* July 1981, p. 45.

Howard, Clinton. "Pharmacological Activities of Aloe Vera Gel." Carrington Laboratories, Irving, TX.

Humes, Edward. "Occupational Health Studied: She Shook Her Clothes Clean of Asbestos and Now Is Ill." *Tucson Citizen Newspaper,* 12 March 1982.

"I've Been Wondering—How Do They Grow Aloe?" *Farm and Ranch Living,* August/September 1982, p. 36.

Johnson, Burt. "Amazing Plant of the Rio Grande Valley." *Rio Grande Valley Edition Supplement to Southwest Farm Press.* Harlingen, TX: Hilltop Gardens.

Kent, Carol Miller. *Aloe Vera.* Arlington, VA: Kent, 1979.

Keough, Carol. "Aloe, the Mystery Medicine." *Organic Gardening,* April 1981, p. 104.

Kolodzey, Jody. "Say 'Aloe'—And Wave Goodbye to Pain." *Prevention,* February 1982, p. 63.

Leung, Albert Y. "Aloe Vera in Cosmetics." *Drug and Cosmetic Industry,* June 1977, p. 34.

———. "The Aloe Vera Mystique." *New York Times Sunday Magazine* (letter to the editor), 6 September 1981, p. 33.

McAnalley, Bill Herman. "The Truth About Aloe." Carrington Laboratories, Irving, TX.

McCauley, R. L., Hing, D. N., Robson, M. C., and Heggers, J. P. "Frostbite Injuries: A Rational Approach Based on the Pathophysiology." *Journal of Trauma,* 23 (2), 1983, p. 143.

McWirker, Norris. *The Dunlop Illustrated Encyclopedia of Facts.* New York: Doubleday, 1969, p. 521.

Meadows, Tim P. "Aloe as a Humectant in New Skin Preparations." *Cosmetics & Toiletries,* 95 (November), 1980, p. 51.

"More on Aloe Vera." *FDA Consumer,* May 1982, p. 2.

Morrow, D. M., Rapaport, M. J., and Strick, R. A. "Hypersensitivity to Aloe." *Archives of Dermatology,* 116 (September), 1980, p. 1064.

National Aloe Science Council. "Analytical and Reporting Procedures and 1983 Program of Work." McLean, VA.

National Aloe Science Council. Brochures: "National Aloe Science Council, Inc." and "Aloe Vera: The Whole Story." McLean, VA.

National Aloe Science Council. *NASC Insight, Quarterly Newsletter,* June
    1984.

Piper, Chuck, and Baxter, Kevin. "Treating Injuries with Aloe Vera." *Runner's
    World,* January 1983, p. 44.

"Placebos Can Be Dangerous To Your Health." *Psychology Today,* 15 (April),
    1981, p. 26.

Raine, T. J., London, M. D., Goluch, L., Heggers, J. P., and Robson,
    M. C. "Antiprostaglandins and Antithromboxantes for Treatment of
    Frostbite." *Surgical Forum American College of Surgeons,* XXXI, 1980,
    p. 557.

Robson, M. C., Jellema, A., Heggers, J. P., and Hagstrom, W. J. "Care of the
    Healed Burn Wound: A Prospective Randomized Study." Abstract from
    paper given at the American Burn Association Twelfth Annual Meeting,
    San Antonio, TX, 27–29 March 1980, p. 94.

Robson, M. C., Heggers, J. P., and Hagstrom, W. J. "Myth, Magic, Witchcraft
    or Fact? Aloe Vera Revisited." *Journal of Burn Care and Rehabilitation,* 3
    (3), May/June 1982, p. 157.

Robson, M. C., Murphy, R. C., and Heggers, J. P. "A New Explanation for the
    Progressive Tissue Loss in Electrical Injuries." *Plastic and Reconstructive
    Surgery,* March 1984, p. 431.

Rudolph, R., and Noe, J. *Chronic Problem Wounds.* Boston: Little Brown,
    1983, p. 34.

"Skin Care Products: A State of the Industry Report." *Drug and Cosmetic In-
    dustry,* September 1984, p. 32.

Skousen, Max B. *The Aloe Vera Handbook.* Huntington Beach, CA: Universal
    Concepts.

——. *Aloe Vera: New Scientific Discoveries.* Cypress, CA: Aloe Vera Research
    Institute, 1982.

——. *The Ancient Egyptian Medicine Plant: Aloe Vera Handbook.* Cypress,
    CA: Aloe Vera Research Institute, 1979, 1982.

——. *Quotations From Medical Journals on Aloe Research.* Cypress, CA: Aloe
    Vera Research Institute.

Smith, D. J., Zachary, L. S., Heggers, J. P., and Robson, M. C. "Pathogenesis of Inadvertent Intra-Arterial Drug Injection Injuries." *Surgical Forum,* 36, October 1985, p. 578.

Smoot, E. C. "The Effects of Anti-Inflammatory Agents on Acute and Late Radiation Skin Changes in the Rat." Discussion presented at the Plastic Surgery Research Council 27th Annual Meeting, 14–17 March, 1982, San Diego, CA.

Smothers, Don L. "Aloe Vera: The Importance of Processing." *Drug & Cosmetic Industry,* January 1983, p. 76.

Southwest Institute for Natural Sources. "Aloe Vera Profile." Grand Prairie, TX.

Taylor-Donald, Laurie. "Aloe Vera: The Wand of Heaven." *Bestways,* August 1980, p. 52.

——. "Aloe Vera—Nature's Miracle." *Bestways,* June 1981, p. 26.

——. "A Runner's Guide to Discovering the Secrets of the Aloe Vera Plant." *Runner's World,* December 1981, p. 38.

——. "Aloe: The Miracle of Aloe Vera." *Fit,* August 1982, p. 70.

Terry Corporation. "Aloe in Brief." Melbourne, FL.

Tisserand, Maggie. *Aromatherapy For Women.* New York: Thorsons Publishers, Inc., 1985.

Tyler, V., Brady, L., and Robbers, J. *Pharmacognosy.* Philadelphia: Lea & Febiger, 1981.

Waller, G. R., Mangiafico, S., and Ritchey, C. R. "A Chemical Investigation of *Aloe barbadensis* Miller." *Proceedings of the Oklahoma Academy of Science,* 58 (June), 1978, p. 69.

Wolfe, Bill, and Iller, Pepper. "Aloe Vera—An Ancient Plant For Modern Dentistry." Pepperdent brochure, Longwood, FL.

Zimmerman, David R. *The Essential Guide to Nonprescription Drugs.* New York: Harper & Row.